Self Assessment in Rheumatology

AF145052

Yousaf Ali

Self Assessment in Rheumatology

An Essential Q & A Study Guide

Second Edition

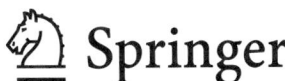 Springer

Yousaf Ali
Mount Sinai Hospital
New York, NY
USA

ISBN 978-3-319-89392-1   ISBN 978-3-319-89393-8   (eBook)
https://doi.org/10.1007/978-3-319-89393-8

Library of Congress Control Number: 2018946140

© Springer International Publishing AG, part of Springer Nature 2018
This work is subject to copyright. All rights are reserved by the Publisher, whether the whole or part of
the material is concerned, specifically the rights of translation, reprinting, reuse of illustrations, recitation,
broadcasting, reproduction on microfilms or in any other physical way, and transmission or information
storage and retrieval, electronic adaptation, computer software, or by similar or dissimilar methodology
now known or hereafter developed.
The use of general descriptive names, registered names, trademarks, service marks, etc. in this publication
does not imply, even in the absence of a specific statement, that such names are exempt from the relevant
protective laws and regulations and therefore free for general use.
The publisher, the authors and the editors are safe to assume that the advice and information in this book
are believed to be true and accurate at the date of publication. Neither the publisher nor the authors or the
editors give a warranty, express or implied, with respect to the material contained herein or for any errors
or omissions that may have been made. The publisher remains neutral with regard to jurisdictional claims
in published maps and institutional affiliations.

Printed on acid-free paper

This Springer imprint is published by the registered company Springer International Publishing AG
part of Springer Nature
The registered company address is: Gewerbestrasse 11, 6330 Cham, Switzerland

Preface

This second edition book is for anyone interested in General Rheumatology or Medicine and should be both fun and educational. It is not intended to be a comprehensive board review but written to stimulate further reading and enjoyment. The cases are real world and reflect a busy inpatient and outpatient consultative practice. I trust the reader will enjoy the mental exercises from both the usual and the unusual cases presented.

I would like to thank my parents and wife for their support in my career and a special thanks to Dr. Margrit Wiesendanger for her careful review of the manuscript. I welcome any comments or criticisms and the responsibility for any errors is mine alone.

New York, NY, USA   Yousaf Ali, MD

Contents

Chapter 1
Questions 1–10

© Springer International Publishing AG, part of Springer Nature 2018
Y. Ali, *Self Assessment in Rheumatology*,
https://doi.org/10.1007/978-3-319-89393-8_1

Question 1

You are asked to assess this 68-year old male patient for vasculitis. He has a history of congestive heart failure, type 2 diabetes and osteoarthritis. Lab tests for viral, infectious causes are negative. He has no antibodies to neutrophil cytoplasmic antigens or nuclear antigens and the Erythrocyte Sedimentation Rate (ESR) is mildly elevated at 57 mm/h.

What is the most likely diagnosis and how would you treat the patient?

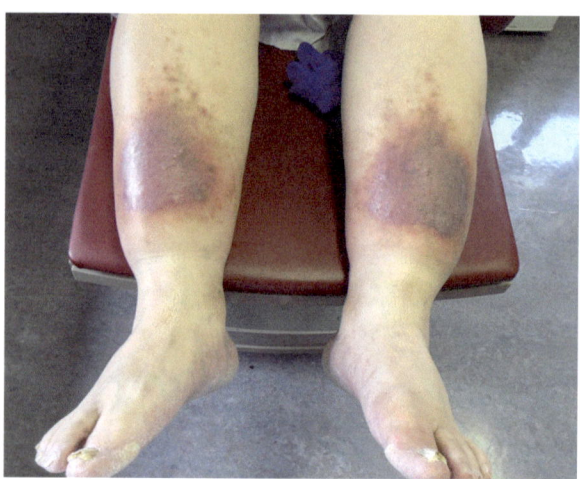

Question 2

A 23-year-old male is referred for evaluation of a three-month history of ankle pain, alternating buttock pain and morning stiffness. He has difficulty ambulating and on exam has enthesopathy of his left Achilles tendon. He has been evaluated by a prior physician due to an elevated ESR of 72 mm/h. What procedure has been performed? What is the most likely result of this procedure?

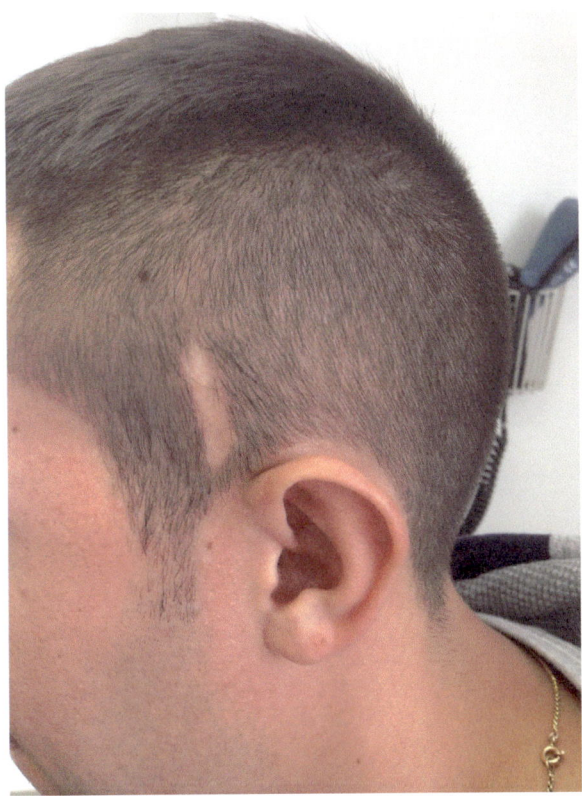

Question 3

A 28-year-old Pakistani female presents with acutely swollen hands. She is a teacher who has difficulty with daily activities, morning stiffness and hand pain for the past eight weeks. She has tender metacarpophalangeal and proximal interphalangeal joints. Her labs reveal a positive anti-cyclic citrullinated antibody (CCP) and rheumatoid factor (RF) but no erosions on radiographs. How would you treat this patient acutely?

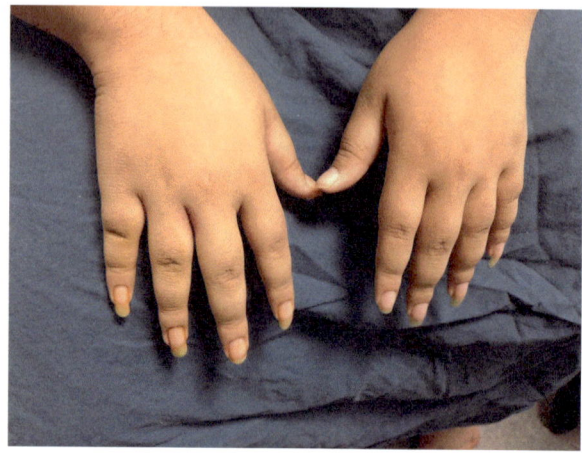

Question 4

This 40-year old female has a history of chronic renal failure and has just completed an MRI with gadolinium to evaluate a breast mass. The MRI result was normal but she has developed skin tightening and chest discomfort. The skin is indurated and has a p'eau d'orange appearance.

What complication has occurred?

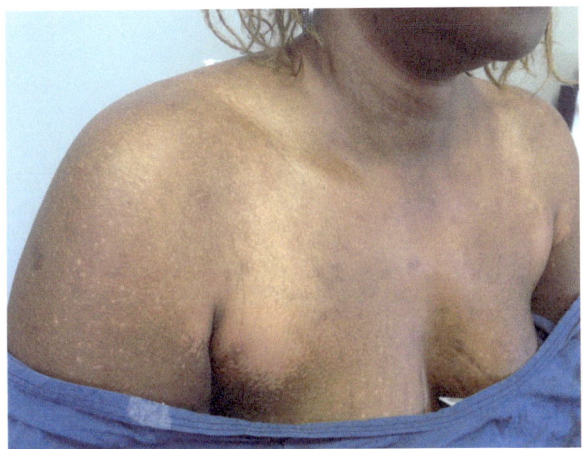

Question 5

This 25-year-old female presents with painful shin lesions. How would you evaluate her and what are the commoner causes?

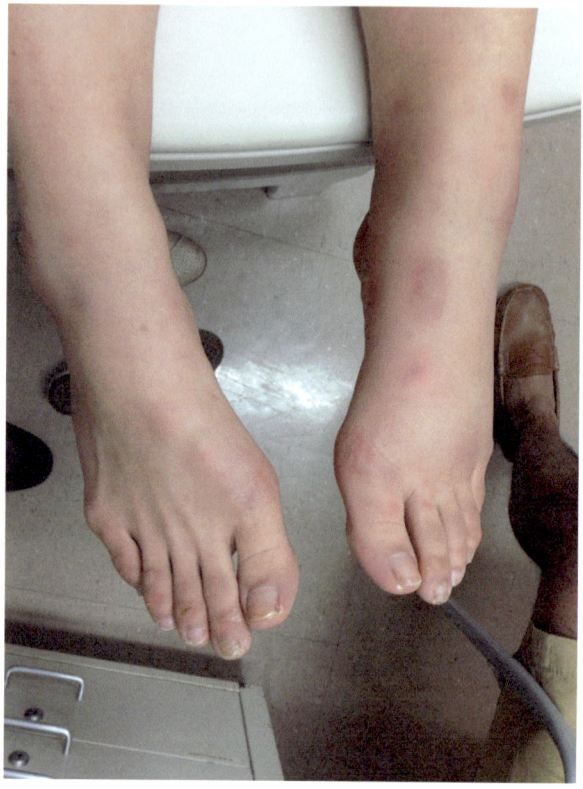

Question 6

This patient has primary Sclerosing Cholangitis (PSC) and chronic diarrhea. What complication has occurred? Discuss management of the skin lesions.

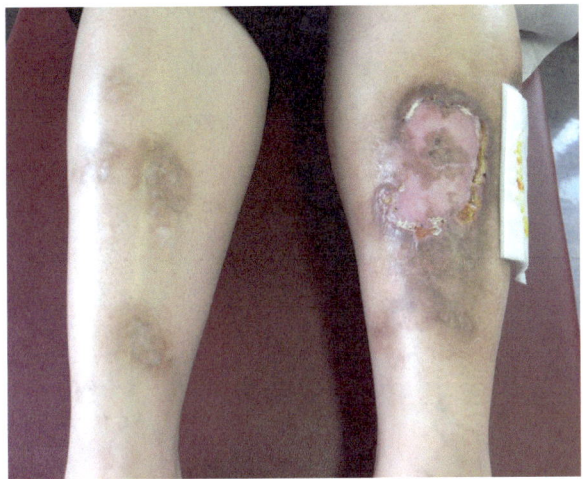

Question 7

This patient has Raynaud's phenomenon and a ten-year history of Dermatomyositis. What findings are noted in the hands? What is the best way to examine this area more closely and what is the differential diagnosis of this finding?

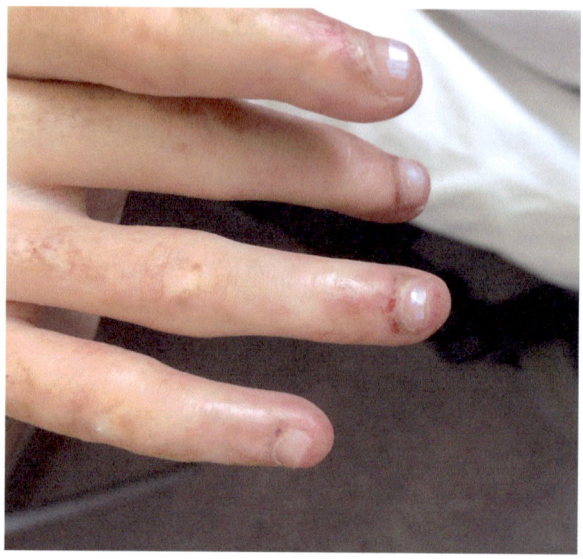

Question 8

A 44-year-old male presents with new onset of lower extremity edema in the context of a rash on his lower extremities and epistaxis. His biopsy result is pending. What diagnoses are you considering?

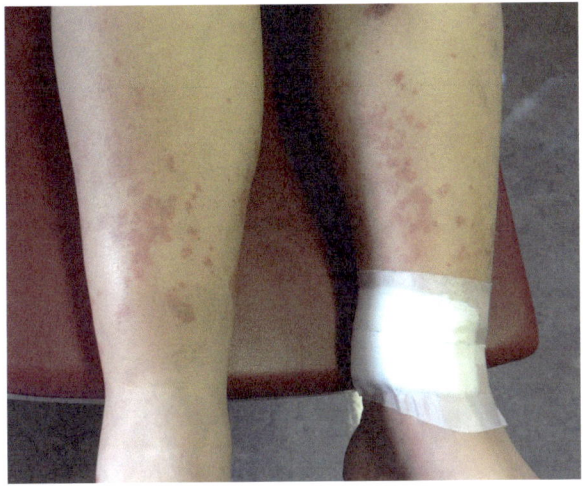

Question 9

This 72-year-old male has a history of chronic tophaceous gout and renal transplantation 10 years previously. He developed Stevens Johnson syndrome on allopurinol and alopecia on febuxostat. How would you treat his deposits?

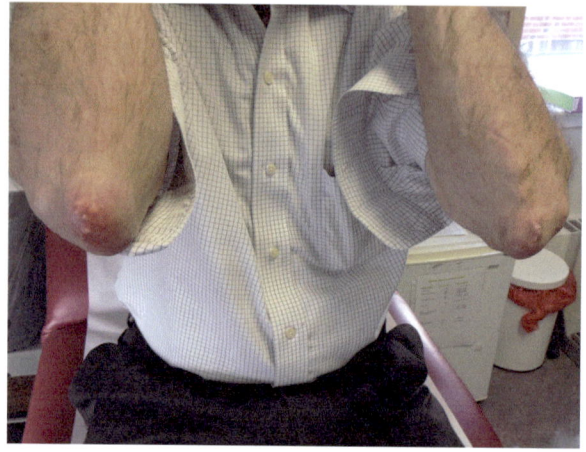

Question 10

This 50-year-old African American female is referred due to bilateral ankle arthritis. What lesions are visible and how does this help the diagnosis? What additional tests are indicated?

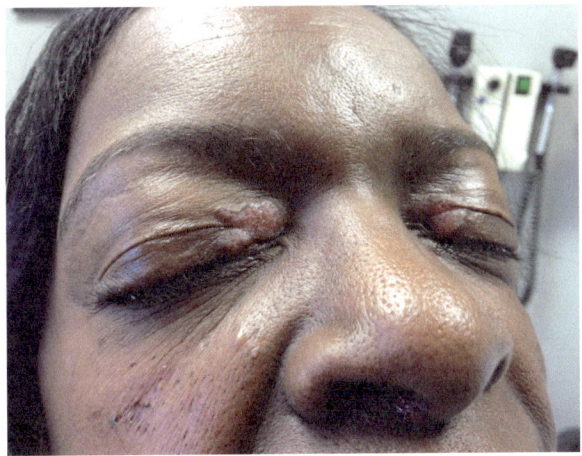

Answer 1: Lipodermatosclerosis

This is unlikely to be vasculitis due to the normal serologies, with indurated, sclerotic plaques which appear "bound down". This is characterized by sclerosing panniculitis on biopsy and is classically associated with an "inverted champagne bottle" appearance [1].

Answer 2

This patient most likely has a Spondyloarthropathy with unilateral Achilles tendonitis, probable sacroiliitis and elevated inflammatory markers. Due to his elevated ESR, he has been sent for a temporal artery biopsy to exclude Giant Cell arteritis (GCA). Since this is a disease of people over the age of 50 with headaches, GCA would be extremely unlikely in this clinical setting. The biopsy yielded negative results and was most likely unnecessary [2, 3].

Answer 3

This patient has a symmetrical small joint arthropathy and antibodies consistent with RA. Her occupational history does raise the issue of an acute parvovirus arthritis but this is less likely given the duration and positive RA serologies. She should be treated with a course of corticosteroids and disease modifying therapy, such as methotrexate or sulfasalazine [4, 5].

Answer 4: Nephrogenic systemic fibrosis (NFS)

NFS is a rare disorder that occurs in some individuals with kidney dysfunction following administration of Gadolinium. This patient has marked areas of induration and hypopigmentation resembling scleroderma. Histologically the lesions are characterized by disorganized bundles of collagen with fibroblast like epithelioid cells or stellate cells. This can occur acutely and may be caused by direct deposition of Gadolinium in the skin [6, 7].

Answer 5: Erythema nodosum (EN)

This patient has erythematous nummular lesions over the shins. Histologically these are most consistent with septal panniculitis and commonly associated with infections such as streptococcus, Tuberculosis, oral contraceptive pills and sulfa containing drugs. As part of the evaluation, autoimmune diseases such as Behcet's, Inflammatory Bowel disease and sarcoidosis should be considered. If appropriate, Pregnancy should be excluded. Even without specific treatment EN often resolves with symptomatic support in many patients [8].

Answer 6: Pyoderma gangrenosum (PG)

This patient most likely has inflammatory bowel disease and inflammation of both intra and extra-hepatic ducts resulting in primary sclerosing cholangitis (PSC). She has developed PG which is a rare ulcerating skin condition that often responds to high dose steroids and Biologic therapy. A skin biopsy is often needed to establish the diagnosis and 50% of patients with PG have a systemic disease such as ulcerative colitis [9].

Answer 7: Dilated nail fold capillaries

Nail fold Capillaroscopy is a useful technique used to differentiate primary from secondary Raynaud's. A drop of grade B immersion oil, mineral oil, or lubricant gel (e.g., K-Y Jelly) is placed proximal to the cuticle. Using an ophthalmoscope or low power microscope evenly arranged capillary loops should be seen arising from the nailbed with a hairpin appearance. In patients with Mixed Connective Tissues Disease, Scleroderma and Polymyositis/Dermatomyositis dilated loops with "dropout" may be seen [10].

Answer 8: Leucocytoclastic vasculitis (LCV)

This patient has a purpuric type rash on the lower extremities which appears consistent with LCV or a hypersensitivity vasculitis. Common causes include medication induced, antiphospholipid syndrome, Behcet's disease, Churg-Strauss syndrome (CSS), granulomatosis with polyangiitis (GPA), Henoch-Schonlein Purpura, urticarial vasculitis, immune thrombocytopenic purpura, and meningococcemia.

Since there is epistaxis either a bleeding disorder or GPA/CSS should be strongly considered [11].

Answer 9

He needs uric acid lowering therapy and options are limited. Uricosuric agents are contraindicated due to his renal dysfunction thus, if available, he should be considered for Pegloticase. This is a mammalian PEGylated uricase that is highly effective at lowering serum uric acid and dissolving tophi. It appears to be well tolerated in renal failure patients [12, 13].

Answer 10: Lupus Pernio

Lupus Pernio is a form of cutaneous Sarcoidosis characterized by raised violaceous lesions over the nose, cheeks and eyes. The term is a misnomer as histologically it is characterized by granulomatous inflammation. A serum calcium, skin biopsy and chest radiograph would be helpful in establishing the diagnosis. Ankle arthritis is a common manifestation of sarcoid arthropathy and should also raise the clinical suspicion [14].

References

1. Keller EC, Tomecki KJ, Alraies MC. Distinguishing cellulitis from its mimics. Cleve Clin J Med. 2012;79(8):547–52.
2. Buttgereit F, Dejaco C, Matteson EL, Dasgupta B. Polymyalgia rheumatica and giant cell arteritis: a systematic review. JAMA. 2016;315(22):2442–58.
3. Rudwaleit M, Taylor WJ. Classification criteria for psoriatic arthritis and ankylosing spondylitis/axial spondyloarthritis. Best Pract Res Clin Rheumatol. 2010;24(5):589–604.
4. Moore L. Parvovirus-associated arthritis. Curr Opin Rheumatol. 2000;12(4):289–94.

5. Smolen JS, Aletaha D, McInnes IB. Rheumatoid arthritis. Lancet. 2016;388(10055):2023–38.
6. Khawaja AZ, Cassidy DB, Shakarchi JA, McGrogan DG, Inston NG, Jones RG. Revisiting the risks of MRI with gadolinium based contrast agents—review of literature and guidelines. Jones Insights Imag. 2015;6(5):553–8.
7. High WA, Ayers RA, Chandler J, et al. Gadolinium is detectable within the tissue of patients with nephrogenic systemic fibrosis. J Am Acad Dermatol. 2007;56(1):21–6.
8. Blake T, Manahan M, Rodins K. Erythema nodosum – a review of an uncommon panniculitis. Dermatol Online. 2014;20(4):22376.
9. Gettler S, Rothe M, Grin C, Grant-Kels J. Optimal treatment of pyoderma gangrenosum. Am J Clin Dermatol. 2003;4(9):597–608.
10. Ingegnoli F, Smith V, Sulli A, Cutolo M. Capillaroscopy in routine diagnostics: potentials and limitations. Curr Rheumatol Rev. 2018;14(1):5–11. https://doi.org/10.2174/15733971136661 70615084229.
11. Micheletti RG, Werth VP. Small vessel vasculitis of the skin. Rheum Dis Clin N Am. 2015;41(1):21–32. vii
12. Baraf SB, Becker MA, Gutierrez-Urena SR, et al. Tophus burden reduction with pegloticase: results from phase 3 randomized trials and open-label extension in patients with chronic gout refractory to conventional therapy Herbert. Arthritis Res Ther. 2013;15(5):R137.
13. Bleyer AJ, Wright D, Alcorn H. Pharmacokinetics and pharmacodynamics of pegloticase in patients with end-stage renal failure receiving hemodialysis. Clin Nephrol. 2015;83(5):286–92.
14. Rao DA, Dellaripa PF. Extrapulmonary manifestations of sarcoidosis. Rheum Dis Clin N Am. 2013;39(2):277–97.

Chapter 2
Questions 11–20

© Springer International Publishing AG, part of Springer Nature 2018
Y. Ali, *Self Assessment in Rheumatology*,
https://doi.org/10.1007/978-3-319-89393-8_2

Question 11

You are asked to see a 28-year-old patient with chronic low back pain of several years duration. A lumbar spine radiograph is performed which is shown below. What key radiographic findings are noted? What is the name of this syndrome and how would you treat the patient?

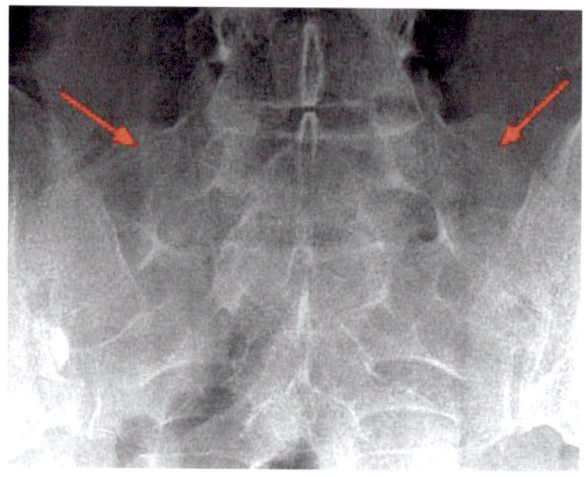

Question 12

You are asked to evaluate a 37-year-old male from Trinidad. He is referred to you due to intermittent toe pain of several months duration. He also admits to weight loss and systemic malaise. His labs are unremarkable apart from an ESR of 65 mm/h and +RF of 108 IU. His joint exam is unremarkable and cardiac exam reveals sinus tachycardia and a 2/6 diastolic murmur at the apex. Retinal exam reveals areas of hemorrhage with pale centers.

What tests are indicated and what is the most likely diagnosis?

Question 13

A 63-year old orthopedic surgeon is evaluated for chronic neck pain. He describes multiple old neck injuries as a medical student playing football. He appears neuro-vascularly intact with preserved strength, power and coordination. Cervical compressive tests are negative and he has no muscle atrophy. His cardiac exam is normal but there are absent breath sounds at the right base. Cervical radiographs show multilevel degenerative changes with hypertrophic spurring and disc disease.

Can you explain his pulmonary findings?

Question 14

You are asked to consult on a 55 year old Caucasian female with proteinuria. She has no known renal disease and is otherwise well apart from mild depression. Physical examination including Blood Pressure (BP) is normal apart from bipedal edema. Her lab data is as follows:

Hb 10.6 g/dl, WBC 4.2, Plt 455, Cr 1.8 mg/dl, BUN 44, 24-h Urine Protein 4 g. ANA +1:160, Sm/RNP/Ds-DNA negative. Complement, CH50, ESR, CRP, ASO are normal. Anti-phospholipase A2 receptor (PLA-2R) antibody is strongly positive. Renal Biopsy is pending.

What is the most likely diagnosis?

Question 15

A 35-year old male hospital employee presents with acute podagra. He has no past medical history and denies a family history of gout. Arthrocentesis of the first metatarsophalangeal joint yields intracellular uric acid crystals. He does not drink alcohol, has no family history of gout, and does not take diuretics. He drinks two cans of soda daily, eats at the hospital cafeteria and eats red meat once per month.

His lab data reveals intact renal and hematologic indices. Serum uric Acid is elevated at 8.9 mg/dl. His BP is 135/80 mm Hg and the rest of his physical examination is unremarkable.

What is the most likely etiology to his gout?

Question 16

A 22-year-old female presents with acute dyspnea and hemoptysis. She has no known past medical history. She denies sick contacts, fever, recent travel or anticoagulants. On examination she is afebrile but tachypneic using her accessory muscles. She has oral ulcerations, a malar rash and arthritis of her left wrist. Cardiac exam reveals sinus tachycardia without jugular venous distension or added heart sounds. She has diffuse bibasilar crepitations and is admitted for observation and treatment. Her CXR shows diffuse hazy infiltrates and she is treated empirically with broad spectrum antibiotics and supportive care. She fails to improve and you are asked to see her on the basis of abnormal labs: Hb 9.5, g/dl MCV 90, Plt 65, WBC 12,000 without left shift. Her metabolic profile is normal and no evidence for bacterial, fungal, viral or mycobacterial organisms are found. ANA is 1:40 dilutions. Anti-double stranded-DNA 55 (elevated), serum complements are normal. Anti-Neutrophil cytoplasmic antibodies (ANCA), RF, anti-CCP antibodies are negative. On day 3 her hemoglobin (Hb) drops to 6 g/dl and she is transferred to the Intensive Care unit.

What is the most likely diagnosis and how would you confirm this? What treatment is indicated and what is the evidence for this?

Question 17

A 28-year-old male presents with marked am stiffness in the back. He has a history of uveitis but no psoriasis, bowel disease or urethritis. His father had reactive Arthritis. On examination, he has a mildly decreased spinal expansion but no sacro-iliac tenderness, synovitis or enthesopathy. Ocular exam confirms anterior uveitis. Labs reveal a C-reactive protein (CRP) of 15 mg/dl but negative RF, CCP antibodies, positive HLA-B27 antigen but normal ESR. His radiographs fail to reveal sacroiliitis or spinal fusion.

   What is the most likely diagnosis and how would you treat this?

Question 18

A 35-year old banker presents with Crohn's disease (CD) presents to the rheumatology clinic with new onset of psoriasis and oligoarthritis. He fails to respond to sulfasalazine and methotrexate and a trial of Secukinumab is undertaken. Six weeks after starting he is hospitalized with acute abdominal pain and diarrhea. What complication has occurred?

Question 19

A 65-year-old female with known postmenopausal osteoporosis is transferred from an outside hospital for severe hip pain. She underwent menopause at age 42 and has taken alendronate for the past decade. Her radiographs are not available for review but the report reveals a fracture 3 cm distal to the lesser trochanter with cortical thickening and a medial cortical beak.

You are asked by orthopedics to evaluate her. What is the most likely diagnosis and etiology?

Question 20

A 77-year-old African American female presents with bilateral refractory cramps in the lower extremities. She has an exercise tolerance of 100 yards and moderate low back pain. Her exam is unrevealing and metabolic profile including electrolytes are normal. She is a non-smoker and ankle brachial indices are normal.

What is the most likely diagnosis and treatment?

Answer 11: Bartoletti's syndrome
This condition is characterized by the presence of a variation of the fifth lumbar (L5) vertebra with a large transverse process, either articulated or fused with the sacral basis or iliac crest, producing a chronic, persistent lower back pain (see red arrows above showing sacralization of transverse processes). Sometimes the pain can be radicular. Treatment is controversial but can include local injections, radio-frequency sensory ablation or surgical resection [1].

Answer 12
This patient has evidence of a systemic vasculitis with embolic phenomena including joint pain and Roth spots. Although the rheumatoid factor is elevated this reflects non-specific B cell stimulation and he does not meet criteria for RA. His cardiac findings are consistent with an insufficiency murmur and probable subacute bacterial endocarditis. Blood cultures and an echocardiogram are indicated [2].

Answer 13: Right phrenic nerve paralysis with elevated hemi diaphragm
This patient has sustained a phrenic nerve damage from prior neck trauma. The absent breath sounds are most likely due to a raised hemi diaphragm from unilateral diaphragmatic nerve paralysis. A chest radiograph (CXR) will confirm this. If this is chronic and the patient is asymptomatic no intervention is warranted [3].

Answer 14: Idiopathic primary membranous nephropathy (IPMN)
Although the differential diagnosis of nephrotic syndrome is broad, the presence of anti-PLA 2 antibodies in patients with nephrotic range proteinuria is highly sensitive and specific for IPMN. PLA2R is expressed on the surface of podocytes and binds soluble phospholipase A2. It is assumed that binding of the autoantibodies to PLA2R results in formation of in situ immune complexes in the area of the glomerular basement membrane. This leads to nephrotic syndrome [4, 5].

Answer 15: High fructose intake from soda
This patient has no traditional risk factors apart from his dietary intake of soda which increases the risk of gout by up to 85%. Fructose is metabolized to uric acid and is prevalent in sugary canned drinks [6].

Answer 16: Diffuse alveolar hemorrhage (DAH)
This patient has Systemic Lupus Erythematosus (SLE) as evidenced by the malar rash, leucopenia, arthritis and positive serologies. She has new onset of pulmonary infiltrates in the context of a sudden drop in the hemoglobin and worsening respiratory function. The most likely scenario in the absence of congestive heart failure or a pulmonary infection is DAH. Paradoxically diffusion capacity in stable patients with a recent hemorrhage is elevated. Since this is life threatening the patient should have bronchoscopy to confirm the diagnosis and then pulse dose intravenous corticosteroids. If the patient has concomitant vasculitis, cytotoxics and plasmapheresis should also be considered [7].

Answer 17: Non-radiographic SpA (Nr-SpA)

This patient has Nr-Spa and meets Criteria for SpondyloArthritis International Society (ASAS) criteria with +HLA-B27 gene in the presence of three SpA features: i.e. uveitis, inflammatory back pain and family history of SpA. Treatment should be commenced with NSAIDs and physical therapy. Escalation to anti-TNF therapy is as indicated [8, 9].

Answer 18: Exacerbation of CD due to secukinumab

Although the mechanism is not clear there have been case reports of exacerbation of disease by anti-IL17A. This cytokine is expressed in the bowel wall of patients with inflammatory bowel disease (IBD) and may be protective. Anti-IL17 blockade appears ineffective in IBD and should be avoided [10, 11].

Answer 19: Sub-trochanteric fracture (STF) due to chronic bisphosphonates

Patients who take oral bisphosphonates for greater than five years have an increased risk of STF and the odds ratio is 2.74. The exact etiology is not clear but most likely due to the suppression of bone remodeling after chronic use. A bisphosphonate holiday should be considered after 5 years [12].

Answer 20: Spinal stenosis

This patient most likely has neurogenic claudication caused by a tight stenotic spinal canal. Anatomically there is narrowing and overgrowth of hypertrophic osteophytes often combined with herniated disc fragments that compress the exiting nerve roots or spinal cord. This results in radicular pain that is exacerbated by ambulation and alleviated by rest. Treatment includes conservative therapy with lifestyle modification, physical therapy, analgesics and epidural injections. Surgery is indicated when there is disabling functional impairment [13].

References

1. Jancuska J, Spivak J, Bendo J. A review of symptomatic lumbosacral transitional vertebrae: Bertolotti's syndrome. Int J Spine Surg. 2015;9:42. https://doi.org/10.14444/2042.
2. Hoen B, Duval X. Infective endocarditis. N Engl J Med. 2013;368:1425–33.
3. Dubé B-P, Dres M, Barnes D. Diaphragm dysfunction: diagnostic approaches and management strategies. J Clin Med. 2016;5(12):113.
4. Dai H, Zhang H, He Y. Diagnostic accuracy of PLA2R autoantibodies and glomerular staining for the differentiation of idiopathic and secondary membranous nephropathy: an updated meta-analysis. Sci Rep. 2015;5:8803.
5. Radice A, Trezzi B, et al. Clinical usefulness of autoantibodies to M-type phospholipase A2 receptor (PLA2R) for monitoring disease activity in idiopathic membranous nephropathy (IMN). Autoimmun Rev. 2016;15(2):146–54.
6. Choi HK, Curhan G. Soft drinks, fructose consumption, and the risk of gout in men: prospective cohort study. BMJ. 2008;336(7639):309–12.

7. Speck U. Diffuse alveolar hemorrhage syndromes. Curr Opin Rheumatol. 2001;13:12–7.
8. Rudwaleit M, van der Heijde D, Landewé R, et al. The assessment of SpondyloArthritis International Society classification criteria for peripheral spondyloarthritis and for spondyloarthritis in general. Ann Rheum Dis. 2011;70(1):25–31.
9. Rudwaleit M. New approaches to diagnosis and classification of axial and peripheral spondyloarthritis. Curr Opin Rheumatol. 2010;22:375–80.
10. Fuss IJ. IL-17: intestinal effector or protector? Mucosal Immunol. 2011;4:366–7.
11. Hueber W, et al. Secukinumab, a human anti-IL-17A monoclonal antibody, for moderate to severe Crohn's disease: unexpected results of a randomized, double-blind placebo-controlled trial. Gut. 2012;61(12):1693–700. https://doi.org/10.1136/gutjnl-2011-301668.
12. Saita Y, Ishijima M, Kaneko K. Atypical femoral fractures and bisphosphonate use: current evidence and clinical implications. Ther Adv Chronic Dis. 2015;6(4):185–93.
13. Genevay S, Atlas SJ. Lumbar spinal stenosis. Best Pract Res Clin Rheumatol. 2010;24(2):253–65.

Chapter 3
Questions 21–30

© Springer International Publishing AG, part of Springer Nature 2018
Y. Ali, *Self Assessment in Rheumatology*,
https://doi.org/10.1007/978-3-319-89393-8_3

Question 21

You are asked to see a 20-year-old Jamaican male who presents with fever and a new right-sided Bell's palsy. On exam, he has uveitis and parotidomegaly but no rash, heart block or stigmata of liver disease. What is the most likely diagnosis?

Question 22

A 54-year-old Japanese female is referred to you from the ophthalmology clinic to evaluate causes of uveitis. She has a history of meningitis and retinal detachment but no inflammatory bowel disease, low back pain or psoriasis. On examination she has vitiligo, low grade fever and meningismus. Her joint exam is normal and there is no evidence of sacroiliitis.

What is the most likely diagnosis and how would you treat her?

Question 23

A 40-year-old obese female accountant presents with right hand coldness with associated parasthesias. She takes no medication and is a non-smoker. Her exam reveals a BMI of 40 with a diminished right radial pulse on inspiration. She is otherwise neurovascularly intact. Her posture is poor and she has enlarged breasts bilaterally. Her apical CXR is normal.

What is the most likely cause of her symptoms?

Question 24

A 19-year-old female college student is seen with recurrent vaginal ulcers. She is sexually active with multiple male partners and does not use barrier protection. An extensive evaluation for sexually transmitted diseases, including syphilis is repeatedly negative. She has no gastrointestinal symptoms and on exam she has multiple shallow vaginal ulcers with painless ulceration of the buccal mucosa. Lab work is drawn and she develops a painful pustule at the site of the venipuncture.

What is the diagnosis?

Question 25

A sixty-six-year old Caucasian male presents with new onset of left sided diplopia and a headache. He has a history of polymyalgia rheumatica and was recently started on ten milligrams of prednisone daily, which he recently tapered to 5 mg. His lab work is unremarkable other than an elevated ESR of 57 mm/h. A brain MRI is normal and physical examination is unremarkable other than left sided optic disc pallor and diplopia with horizontal gaze. A 0.2 cm left temporal artery biopsy is obtained which is reported as having no active arteritis. One week later he loses vision in his left eye.

What complication has occurred and why?

Question 26

You follow a 50 year-old female with known granulomatosis with polyangiitis (GPA). She initially presented with biopsy proven pauci-immune glomerulonephritis that was treated with oral cyclophosphamide and prednisone for 1 year. She has recently transitioned to azathioprine when she presents with new onset of nasal congestion, proptosis and left sided frontal headache. Her examination revealed ocular chemosis, a left sixth cranial nerve palsy and sinus tenderness.

What is the most likely scenario?

Question 27

A 26-year-old male is referred for evaluation of hand pain. His past history includes Pierre Robin Syndrome and deafness. On examination he has multiple neck scars consistent with corrective surgery and bilateral hearing aids. His hands reveal Heberdens and Bouchards nodes but no palpable synovitis.

What is the diagnosis?

Question 28

A 60-year-old female with severe RA presents with the new onset of inability to extend her right 3–5th digits. Palpation of the extensor tendons suggests that they are intact. Her examination reveals synovitis of the metacarpophalangeal joints, both elbows and multiple extensor nodules.

What is the most likely diagnosis?

Question 29

A patient with membranous nephropathy who has been on mycophenylate mofetil (MMF), low dose prednisone and cyclosporine for 5 years, presents with the oral lesions below. What complication has occurred? How would you treat her?

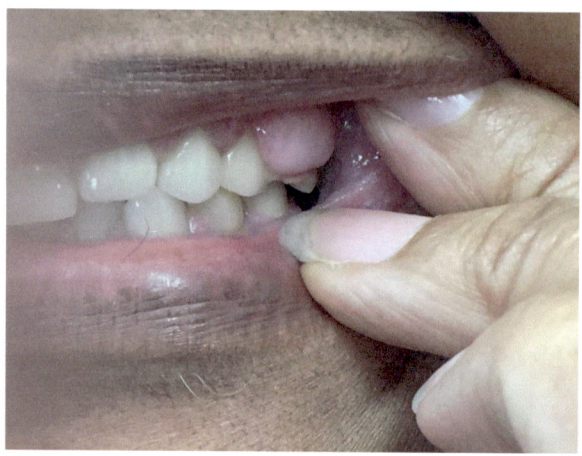

Question 30

The emergency room calls you to see a 30-year-old woman with a distant history of idiopathic thrombotic purpura (ITP). She presents with new onset of pleuritic chest pain. Examination shows a female in mild distress with normal vital signs other than sinus tachycardia. No rubs are heard. She is afebrile but has diminished breath sounds at the left base and is taking shallow breaths. An ECG reveals sinus tachycardia and CXR shows a small left pleural effusion. A Computed Tomographic Angiogram (CTA scan) of the chest showed no evidence for a pulmonary embolus. Laboratory tests reveal normal complete blood count, hepatic and renal function. Old records reveal antibodies to nuclear antigens, Smith and double stranded DNA. Serial cardiac enzymes are negative.

What is the most likely diagnosis and how would you treat her?

Answer 21: Heerfordt's syndrome
Heerfordt's syndrome, also called uveoparotid fever, is characterized by the presence of parotid gland enlargement, facial nerve palsy, anterior uveitis, and fever. This is rare and occurs in about 0.3% of patients with sarcoidosis. The fever and compressive nerve lesion is thought to be due to granulomatous inflammation [1, 2].

Answer 22: Vogt-Koyanagi-Harada syndrome (VKH)
VKH is a rare multisystem inflammatory disorder characterized by panuveitis with serous retinal detachments, and it is often associated with neurologic and cutaneous manifestations, including headache, hearing loss, vitiligo and poliosis. Treatment is usually with high dose oral steroids followed by steroid sparing agents in refractory patients [3].

Answer 23: Thoracic Outlet syndrome (TOS)
This is a controversial condition characterized by compression of the neurovascular bundle at the scalene triangle, costoclavicular and retropectoralis minor spaces. Since compression of both the nerve and artery can occur the patient can present with either neurologic symptoms or hand ischemia. Other features include painless wasting of intrinsic hand muscles, paresthesia, and pain. A careful and detailed medical history and physical examination are the most important diagnostic tools for proper identification of TOS [4].

Answer 24: Behcet's disease (BD)
BD is a multisystem inflammatory disease characterized by recurrent orogenital ulcers with skin lesions that include erythema nodosum, uveitis, CNS, gastrointestinal and joint involvement. Pathergy occurs at the site of skin irritation and is associated with pustule formation. Although the exact mechanisms underlying pathergy are unknown, skin injury caused by needle prick apparently triggers a cutaneous inflammatory response which is much more prominent and extensive than that seen in normal skin. This suggests an increased or aberrant release of cytokines from keratinocytes or other cells in the epidermis or dermis resulting in perivascular infiltration observed on skin biopsy.

   Treatment of BD includes colchicine, NSAIDs, steroids, immunosuppressive therapy and newer biologic agents including anti-TNF therapy [5].

Answer 25: Giant cell arteritis (GCA)
Approximately 10% of patients with PMR develop GCA. This is a large vessel vasculitis characterized by headaches, jaw claudication and scalp tenderness. Ocular lesions occur due to occlusion or vasculitis of various ophthalmic arteries and their branches. Anterior ischemic optic neuropathy (AION) is the most common lesion, which results in optic atrophy and irreversible visual loss. The blindness is usually painless and sudden in onset, thus early recognition of the symptoms is important. Prompt treatment can abort the visual loss. A >2 cm biopsy is ideal as GCA is a disease of discontinuity and skip lesions. In this case the 0.2 cm biopsy is inadequate to exclude the diagnosis in a patient with a moderate pretest probability [6–8].

Answer 26: Cavernous sinus thrombosis

The syndrome results in involvement of extraocular muscles, compression of the trigeminal nerve and frequently extension to involve the optic nerve. The presence of proptosis, with swelling of eyelids and chemosis suggests mass effect within the orbit. Potential causes include traumatic craniomaxillofacial injuries, tumors of the orbit (lymphoma or rhabdomyosarcoma) and adjacent structures. Infection, inflammatory disorders, and vasculitis including GPA are also reported etiologies [9].

Answer 27: Stickler syndrome

Stickler syndrome is a connective tissue disorder that occurs due to mutations in the collagen genes COL11A1, COL11A2 and COL2A1.

Findings include myopia, cataract, and retinal detachment. In some individuals, hearing loss, midfacial underdevelopment and cleft palate can occur either alone or as part of the Pierre-Robin sequence. Rheumatologists may encounter these patients due to precocious osteoarthritis [10].

Answer 28: Entrapment of the posterior interosseous nerve (PIN) at the elbow

The radial nerve branches into its sensory and motor branches at the level of the radiocapitellar joint at the elbow. The PIN is the distal, motor branch of the radial nerve and is susceptible to compression by synovitis at the level of the elbow joint in rheumatoid arthritis. Posterior interosseous nerve (PIN) entrapment is a rare complication of rheumatoid arthritis (RA) which, together with extensor tendon rupture and metacarpophangeal joint dislocation, should be considered in the differential diagnosis of inability to extend the fingers. Clinically, there is sparing of muscles innervated by the radial nerve proximal to the takeoff of the PIN and thus patients lack metacarpophalangeal extension and are only able to weakly extend the wrist with radial deviation. The symptoms often respond favorably to systemic control of the RA [11].

Answer 29: Cyclosporin (CsA) induced gingival hyperplasia

This is an iatrogenic disorder caused by cumulative use of CsA.

For patients who need the drug this can be minimized by elimination of local irritants, meticulous oral hygiene and gingivectomy as needed [12].

Answer 30: Systemic lupus erythematosus (SLE)

This patient has a history of low platelets with new onset serositis, antibodies to nuclear, Smith antigens and double stranded DNA. She meets 2012 SLICC Classification criteria for SLE and she can be treated initially with oral anti-inflammatory medications including NSAIDs or corticosteroids [13].

References

1. Fujiwara K, Furuta Y, Fukuda S. Two cases of Heerfordt's syndrome: a rare manifestation of sarcoidosis. Case Rep Otolaryngol. 2016;2016:3642735.
2. Darlington P, Tallstedt L, Padyukov L, et al. HLA-DRB1* alleles and symptoms associated with Heerfordt's syndrome in sarcoidosis. Eur Respir J. 2011;38(5):1151–7.
3. Sakata VM, da Silva FT, Hirata CE, de Carvalho JF, Yamamoto JH. Diagnosis and classification of Vogt-Koyanagi-Harada disease. Autoimmun Rev. 2014;13(4-5):550–5.
4. Hooper TL, et al. Thoracic outlet syndrome: a controversial clinical condition. Part 1: anatomy, and clinical examination/diagnosis. J Manual Manipulative Ther. 2010;182:74–83.
5. Rokutanda R, Kishimoto M, Okada M. Update on the diagnosis and management of Behçet's disease. Open Access Rheumatol Res Rev. 2015;7:1–8.
6. Weyand CM, Goronzy JJ. Giant-cell arteritis and polymyalgia rheumatica. N Engl J Med. 2014;371(1):50–7.
7. Haering M, Holbro A, Todorova MG, et al. Incidence and prognostic implications of diplopia in patients with giant cell arteritis. J Rheumatol. 2014;41(7):1562–4.
8. Ypsilantis E, Courtney ED, Chopra N, et al. Importance of specimen length during temporal artery biopsy. Br J Surg. 2011;98(11):1556–60.
9. Bone I, Hadley DM. Syndromes of the orbital fissure, cavernous sinus, cerebello- pontine angle, and skull base. J Neurol Neurosurg Psychiatry. 2005;76:iii29–38.
10. Robin NH, Moran RT, Ala-Kokko L. Stickler syndrome. In: Adam MP, Ardinger HH, Pagon RA, et al., editors. GeneReviews®. Seattle, WA: University of Washington; 1993–2017.
11. Malipeddi A, Reddy VR, Kallarackal G. Posterior interosseous nerve palsy: an unusual complication of rheumatoid arthritis: case report and review of the literature. Semin Arthritis Rheum. 2011;40(6):576–9.
12. Aral CA, Dilber E, Aral K, Sarica Y, Sivrikoz ON. Management of cyclosporine and nifedipine-induced gingival hyperplasia. J Clin Diagn Res. 2015;9(12):ZD12–5.
13. Petri M, Orbai AM, Alarcón GS, et al. Derivation and validation of the systemic lupus international collaborating clinics classification criteria for systemic lupus erythematosus. Arthritis Rheum. 2012;64(8):2677–86.

Chapter 4
Questions 31–40

© Springer International Publishing AG, part of Springer Nature 2018
Y. Ali, *Self Assessment in Rheumatology*,
https://doi.org/10.1007/978-3-319-89393-8_4

Question 31

A 45-year old with a distant history of granulomatosis with polyangiitis (GPA) presents with frank hematuria. His prior treatment included oral cyclophosphamide for 2 years and intermittent prednisone. He has no abdominal pain or history of renal stones. His urinalysis confirms non-glomerular hematuria.

What is the most likely complication?

Question 32

A 60-year old African male with tophaceous gout is referred for pegloticase therapy. Soon after his infusion he develops fatigue, dyspnea and dark urine. His laboratory examination reveals feature of hemolytic anemia with an undetectable haptoglobin, macrocytic anemia and elevated LDH. His Methhemoglobin level was 8%, with normal O2 saturation of 99% on room air.

What complication has occurred?

Question 33

An 80-year-old female has refractory left shoulder pain. She has limited range of motion in all planes and cannot abduct past 90°. Analgesics have not helped and she has increased pain with physical therapy. Her radiograph is below.

What is the most likely diagnosis and how would you treat her?

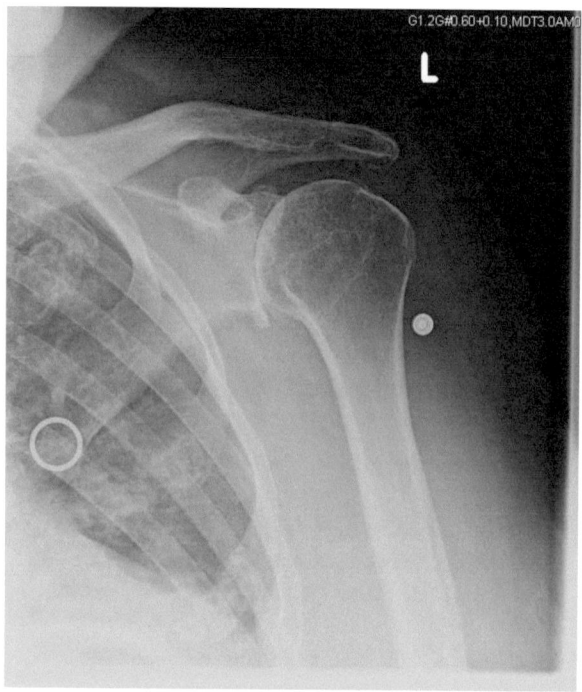

Question 34

A 44-year old female originally from the Philippines, presents with new onset of blurry vision without headaches, diplopia, dizzy spells or accompanying neurologic symptoms. Her ophthalmic examination revealed "bilateral retinal vasculitis" without optic neuritis. She is referred to the rheumatology clinic for evaluation of a systemic disease. Her review of systems and physical examination is normal. Serologic examination reveals high titer ANA 1:2560 titer with antibodies to Smith, RNP, double stranded-DNA and SS-A. Serum complements, renal, hepatic and hematologic indices are normal. Urine does not reveal an active sediment.

She is placed on high dose steroids, 60 mg prednisone daily by her ophthalmologist. One week later her husband calls to inform you of a significant personality change, with delusional behavior.

What is the differential diagnosis and how would you investigate this?

Question 35

A 66-year old white male with a 25-year history of SLE presents with new onset of right knee pain and chronic discoloration on the legs. His regimen includes weekly low dose Methotrexate, Prednisone 5 mg daily and Hydroxychloroquine 400 mg daily. On examination, he has a swollen right knee with fullness in the popliteal fossa and tenderness in the calf. He has been taking the above regimen for over 5 years.

What is the most likely cause of his lesions?

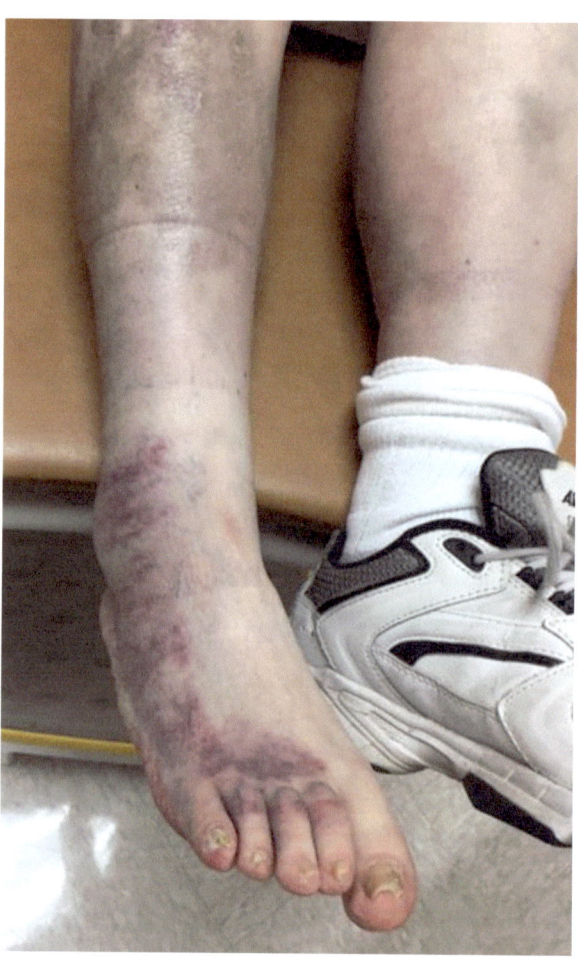

Question 36

A 37-year-old female presents with recurrent pregnancy loss at week 8, 6 and 10. Her obstetrician describes her uterus as arcuate and having a thin lining. As part of her evaluation, serologic testing reveals a low titer anticardiolipin antibody (ACA), negative beta 2-glycoprotein 1(B2 GP1) and negative lupus anticoagulant. These levels do not change with repeat testing after twelve weeks. She has no symptoms and has no history of thrombotic episodes, migraines or livedo. Her ANA is negative and she has a normal complete blood count (CBC) without thrombocytopenia.

Does this patient have the antiphospholipid syndrome (APS)?

Question 37

A 30-year old female has moderately symptomatic Raynaud's disease without extremity ulceration. Symptoms have persisted despite protective measures and may be triggered by stress. Evaluation for secondary causes including hypercoagulability and primary autoimmune diseases, is negative. Her systolic blood pressure (BP) is 90 mmHg and she refuses any topical or oral medications.

   What treatment would you suggest?

Question 38

A 45-year-old female presents with recurrent Achilles tendinopathy that does not respond to physical therapy. She has no clear overuse or rheumatologic diagnosis. On examination you note tenderness at the insertion of the tendon and abnormal nailbed exam. See below.

What is the most likely diagnosis? What else causes this condition?

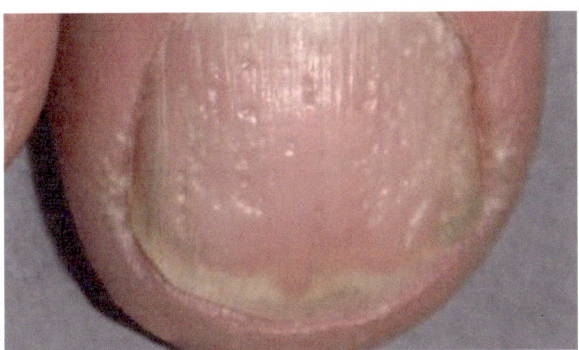

Question 39

A 61-year old female with chronic deforming RA presents with new onset of ocular pain. She was recently started on treatment for osteoporosis and her current regimen includes low dose methotrexate, prednisone and alendronate. What complication has occurred?

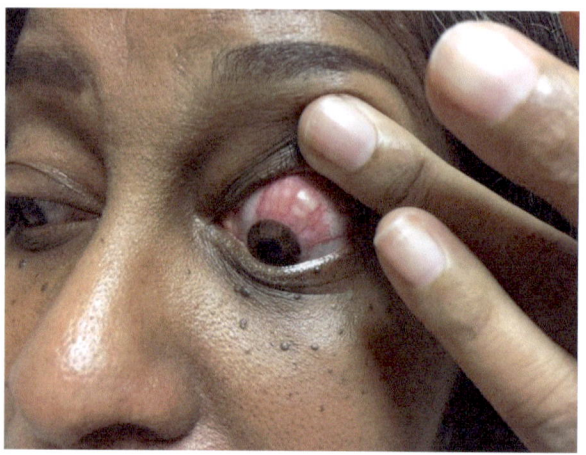

Question 40

A 66-year old male from Panama presents with new onset ankle and wrist arthritis of 2 weeks duration. He has a past history of Type 2 diabetes and hypertension. He denies sick contacts but has had a low-grade fever and mild sore throat. He is not sexually active and has no prior history of joint pain. On examination he has synovitis of his left ankle and right wrist. He has no tophi but has an erythematous rash over his upper arm which appears annular with central fading. Cardiac exam reveals a mitral murmur of insufficiency. He has a low-grade fever and systolic hypertension. Abdominal exam and neurologic exam are normal. After three days in the hospital he develops myoclonus and dysarthria. Laboratory testing reveals a normal metabolic profile, anemia of chronic disease with a markedly elevated ESR of 92 mm/h. Urinalysis is unremarkable. Synovial fluid analysis of the ankle revealed 18,000 nucleated cells without crystals. Joint fluid cultures are negative. A CXR shows mild cardiomegaly. An echocardiogram confirms calcified aortic and mitral valves with moderate mitral valve insufficiency. EKG shows first degree heart block. Brain MRI is normal.

What is the most likely diagnosis and what further tests are indicated?

Answer 31: Cyclophosphamide (CYC) induced transitional cell cancer
CYC can result in toxicity of the urinary bladder resulting in both hemorrhagic cystitis and bladder cancer. In addition to its effect on the bladder, like many other immunosuppressive agents, it has been associated with teratogenicity, infections, sterility and secondary hematologic malignancy. CYC is metabolized by the Cytochrome P450 route to acrolein which accumulates in the bladder and may be one of the causative agents in bladder cancer. Ensuring adequate hydration and consideration of concomitant MESNA administration given orally during CYC treatment is protective [1, 2].

Answer 32: Methemoglobinemia and hemolysis due to G6PD deficiency
Pegloticase can cause severe hemolysis and methemoglobinaemia in glucose-6-phosphate dehydrogenase-deficient individuals. The drug is a pegylated urate oxidase which converts uric acid to water soluble allantoin, this rapidly lowers uric acid. Adverse events may result from this conversion, due to oxidative stress induced by the production of large amounts of hydrogen peroxide (H_2O_2). All patients should be screened prior to starting the drug [3–5].

Answer 33: Left glenohumeral joint osteoarthritis
This patient's radiograph shows narrowing of the glenohumeral joint with osteophytes and subchondral sclerosis. Unfortunately, there are no proven therapies that reverse osteoarthritis (OA) and treatment revolves around maintenance of function and alleviation of pain. Analgesic therapy with NSAIDs or pain relievers such as acetaminophen are the mainstay of treatment. In patients with severe pain a local intraarticular steroid can be considered or else surgical intervention with total shoulder arthroplasty. Given the patient's advanced age, surgical repair should be a last resort [6, 7].

Answer 34: Corticosteroid induced psychosis vs. lupus cerebritis
This patient has serologic evidence of Systemic Lupus Erythematosus (SLE), and retinal vasculitis is a rare ocular complication. The most likely reason for the sudden change in mental status is steroid induced psychosis. This occurs in a small percentage of patients on steroids and appears dose dependent and early on in the treatment course. Since SLE can also affect the brain, an MRI or spinal fluid analysis may be considered to exclude CNS cerebritis or an infection, which is less likely [8, 9].

Answer 35: Ruptured Baker's cyst with crescent sign and hydroxychloroquine (HCQ) toxicity
His skin is chronically discolored which is a sign of chronic HCQ deposition. He also has areas of fresh hemorrhage along the lateral aspect of the foot with clinical evidence of a ruptured popliteal (Baker's) cyst. This is called the crescent sign and suggests hemorrhage down the fascial planes. An ultrasound should be obtained to exclude a deep vein thrombosis (DVT) which can present in a similar fashion [10–12].

Answer 36

According to the revised International Criteria for APS, patients must have recurrent arteriovenous thrombosis or unexplained pregnancy loss before the tenth week of gestation in the absence of maternal anatomic, chromosomal or hormonal abnormalities. This should occur in the presence of medium titer anticardiolipin/B2 Microglobulin antibodies or lupus anticoagulant positivity at least 12 weeks apart. Since this patient has only a low titer ACA and a maternal reason for pregnancy loss she does not meet criteria for APS. No long term anticoagulation is indicated [13].

Answer 37: Biofeedback

Raynaud's disease is characterized by intermittent peripheral vasoconstriction leading to pallor, cyanosis and reactive vasodilation of the arterioles of fingers and toes. Since her BP is low and she is reluctant to take medications traditional agents such as calcium channel blockers or topical nitrates cannot be used. Psychological intervention, including biofeedback, may have a role in this patient. Biofeedback involving relaxation techniques, guided imagination, and in parallel, computer-assisted monitoring of sympathetic arousal, has been reported to lead to symptom reduction as a unique treatment or in conjunction with other treatment modalities [14].

Answer 38: Psoriatic arthritis (PsA)

This patient has nail pitting and enthesopathy which raises the possibility of PsA. Nail pitting also occurs in lichen planus, alopecia areata, eczema and reactive arthritis. A more detailed look for psoriatic lesions including the scalp, navel, sub mammary region and gluteal folds should be undertaken. Although NSAIDs are often effective, if the arthritis remains active, local glucocorticoid injections can be considered followed by a biologic agent such as a TNF inhibitor. Non-biologic DMARDs have not been shown to be effective in enthesopathy or dactylitis [15–17].

Answer 39: Bisphosphonate (BP) induced scleritis

Since this patient has stable RA and was recently introduced to an oral bisphosphonate this appears the most likely culprit. Scleritis is a rare but well recognized complication of BP therapy. The mechanism is unclear, but it may be related to secretion of the drug into the lacrimal glands and irritation of the mucous membranes. Prompt removal of the drug and local anti-inflammatory agents usually result in complete resolution [18].

Answer 40: Acute rheumatic fever (ARF)

This patient meets criteria for ARF with four major criteria (carditis, polyarthritis, chorea, erythema marginatum) and two minor criteria (fever, elevated acute phase reactants). An echocardiogram, blood, throat cultures and rapid antigen test should be obtained in addition to antibody testing (ASO test, antistreptococcal DNAse B test) [19, 20].

References

1. Pedersen-Bjergaard J, Ersboll J, Hansen VL, Sorensen BL, Christoffersen K, Hou-Jensen K, et al. Carcinoma of the urinary bladder after treatment with cyclophosphamide for non-Hodgkin's lymphoma. N Engl J Med. 1988;318:1028–32.
2. Monach PA, Arnold LM, Merkel PA. Incidence and prevention of bladder toxicity from cyclophosphamide in the treatment of rheumatic diseases: a data-driven review. Arthritis Rheum. 2010;62(1):9–21.
3. Owens RE, Swanson H, Twilla JD. Hemolytic anemia induced by pegloticase infusion in a patient with G6PD deficiency. J Clin Rheumatol. 2016;22(2):97–8.
4. Geraldino-Pardilla L, Sung D, Xu JZ, et al. Methaemoglobinaemia and haemolysis following pegloticase infusion for refractory gout in a patient with a falsely negative glucose-6-phosphate dehydrogenase deficiency result. Rheumatology. 2014;53(12):2310–1.
5. Sonbol MB, Yadav H, Vaidya R, Rana V, Witzig TE. Methemoglobinemia and hemolysis in a patient with G6PD deficiency treated with rasburicase. Am J Hematol. 2013;88(2):152–4.
6. Boyd AD Jr, Thornhill TS. Surgical treatment of osteoarthritis of the shoulder. Rheum Dis Clin N Am. 1988;14:591.
7. Rispoli DM, Sperling JW, Athwal GS, et al. Humeral head replacement for the treatment of osteoarthritis. J Bone Joint Surg Am. 2006;88:2637.
8. Md N, Kalthum U, Zahidin AZA, Yong TK. Retinal vasculitis in systemic lupus erythematosus: an indication of active disease. Clin Pract. 2012;2(2):e54.
9. Kenna HA, Poon AW, de los Angeles CP, Koran LM. Psychiatric complications of treatment with corticosteroids: review with case report. Psychiatry Clin Neurosci. 2011;65:549–60. https://doi.org/10.1111/j.1440-1819.2011.
10. Berkun Y, et al. A man with swollen calf and discoloration of the foot. Postgrad Med J. 2002;78:304.
11. Kraag G, Thevathasan EM, Gordon DA, Walker IH. The hemorrhagic crescent sign of acute synovial rupture. Ann Intern Med. 1976;85:477.
12. Puri PK, Lountzis NI, Tyler W, Ferringer T. Hydroxychloroquine-induced hyperpigmentation: the staining pattern. J Cutan Pathol. 2008;35(12):1134–7.
13. Ruiz-Irastorza G, Crowther M, Branch W, Khamashta MA. Antiphospholipid syndrome. Lancet. 2010;376(9751):1498–509.
14. Karavidas MK, Tsai PS, Yucha C, McGrady A, Lehrer PM. Thermal biofeedback for primary Raynaud's phenomenon: a review of the literature. Appl Psychophysiol Biofeedback. 2006;31(3):203–16.
15. Orbai A-M, Weitz J, Siegel EL, et al. Systematic review of treatment effectiveness and outcome measures for enthesitis in psoriatic arthritis. J Rheumatol. 2014;41:2290–4.
16. Rose S, Toloza S, Bautista-Molano W, et al. GRAPPA Dactylitis Study Group. Comprehensive treatment of dactylitis in psoriatic arthritis. J Rheumatol. 2014;41:2295–300.
17. Richert B, Caucanas M, André J. Diagnosis using nail matrix. Dermatol Clin. 2015;33(2):243–55.
18. Clark EM, Durup D. Inflammatory eye reactions with bisphosphonates and other osteoporosis medications: what are the risks? Ther Adv Musculoskelet Dis. 2015;7(1):11–6.
19. Special Writing Group of the Committee on Rheumatic Fever, Endocarditis, and Kawasaki Disease of the Council on Cardiovascular Disease in the Young of the American Heart Association. Guidelines for the diagnosis of rheumatic fever Jones criteria. JAMA. 1992;268(15):2069–73.
20. Gewitz MH, Baltimore RS, Tani LY, et al. American Heart Association Committee on Rheumatic Fever, Endocarditis, and Kawasaki Disease of the Council on Cardiovascular Disease in the Young. Revision of the Jones criteria for the diagnosis of acute rheumatic fever in the era of Doppler echocardiography: a scientific statement from the American Heart Association. Circulation. 2015;131(20):1806–18.

Chapter 5
Questions 41–50

© Springer International Publishing AG, part of Springer Nature 2018
Y. Ali, *Self Assessment in Rheumatology*,
https://doi.org/10.1007/978-3-319-89393-8_5

Question 41

A 19-year old Marine falls off a training wall and feels a tear in the shoulder. He presents with pain and increased passive external rotation. He has a positive lift off test, with weakness lifting the internally rotated hand away from the patient's mid lumbar spine.

Which rotator cuff muscle is involved?

Question 42

A 42-year old male presents with recurrent podagra. He has a strong family history of gout but is unable to tolerate colchicine or NSAIDs. Aspiration of the first metatarsophalangeal joint is attempted without success. His serum uric acid is elevated at 9.5 mg/dl. He is reluctant to commence chronic urate lowering therapy and a baseline radiograph is normal.

Are there any other imaging modalities to prove the presence of urate arthritis?

Question 43

A 29-year old pre-menopausal female presents with severe recurrent low back and radicular pain that is associated with her menses. Her past medical history includes pneumothorax. Her weight has remained stable and she has no history of spinal trauma, fever, rash or morning stiffness. Her physical exam is unremarkable other that mild suprapubic pain. She is distally neurovascularly intact. Imaging studies of the spine and pelvis are normal.

What is the most likely diagnosis?

Question 44

A 33-year old female with a history of Crohn's disease affecting the small bowel is referred to rheumatology for new onset incapacitating joint pain. She has previously taken a variety of medications including mesalamine, methotrexate, 6-mercaptopurine, adalimumab and infliximab with varied success but no joint pain. Three months prior to her current presentation, she was started on vedolizumab.

On examination, she has tenderness at the right sacroiliac joint, bilateral Achilles enthesopathy and new onset of uveitis.

Why is her arthritis active?

Question 45

An 80-year-old female is referred to evaluate osteoporosis. She has a declining T score of < -4.5 standard deviations from the mean. She is 30 years post-menopause and did not take estrogen replacement. She took alendronate for 5 years but was recently transitioned to teriperatide due to declining bone mass. Evaluations for secondary causes of osteoporosis were negative. In particular she had no endocrinopathy, hypercalciuria, myeloma or malabsorption. Vitamin D was replete. After 6 months of taking teriperatide her alkaline phosphatase (ALP) was noted to be three times normal.

Discuss.

Question 46

You are asked to see a 55-year old female inpatient who complains of diffuse weakness and the referring team is concerned about a rheumatologic cause. Her symptoms are worse at the end of the day and associated with a change in her voice like "Donald Duck". She has a history of vitiligo and hyperthyroidism. On examination, she has bilateral ptosis and mild dysphonia. Her muscle strength is 5/5 all groups and laboratory tests including CPK are normal.

What is the most likely diagnosis?

Question 47

You are asked to evaluate a 79-year old female with recurrent pneumonia and RA. She is admitted with a fever and local infiltrate on CXR. Due to diffuse basilar crackles, a high-resolution CT scan is obtained.

What does this show and what is the etiology of her recurrent infections?

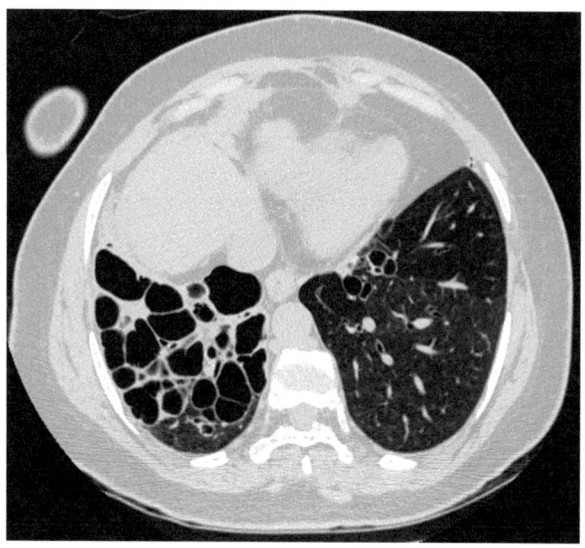

Question 48

A 43-year old female is admitted with severe low back pain and radicular pain. On examination, she has loss of sensation of the dorsum of the right foot and weakness with toe dorsiflexion. Straight leg raising reproduces pain at 30° and she has mild right thigh weakness.

What is the involved nerve root?

Question 49

A 70-year old female with chronic RA is admitted with new onset dyspnea. She has a history of stable myelodysplastic syndrome. She is maintained on oral methotrexate and low dose prednisone for the past 10 years without dose changes. She has not traveled and has no fever or productive sputum. On examination, she is in moderate distress with bilateral lower zone crepitations and centrally cyanosed. There is no jugular venous distension or third heart sound. Her laboratory tests are unremarkable other than slight elevation of LDH. Her CXR showed hazy diffuse infiltrates and CT scan is shown below. Bronchoalveolar lavage (BAL) revealed negative bacterial, viral and mycobacterial cultures. Urinary and serum tests for atypical pneumonia were negative. The BAL fluid appeared opaque with abundant periodic acid-Schiff positive extracellular material.

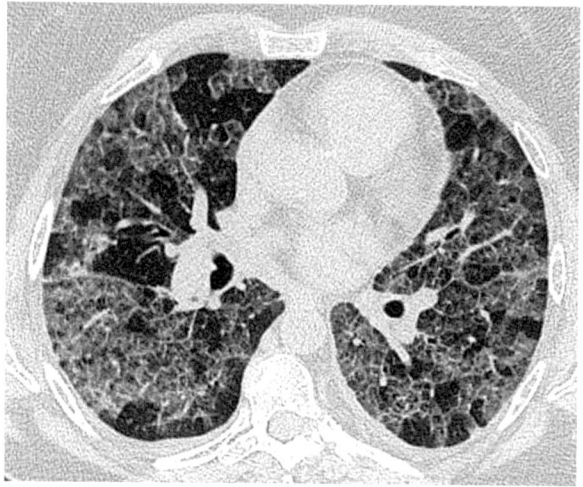

What is the Diagnosis and what does the CT show?

Question 50

A 24-year old female presents with inspiratory chest pain, arthritis and fatigue. She has no past history and takes no medications. Her physical examination reveals the following: BP 102/80, Pulse 114, respiratory Rate 22, temperature 98.4 °F. conjunctival pallor with mild scleral icterus, sinus tachycardia and a right pleural rub. She has polysynovitis of the hands, wrists and elbows but no organomegaly or abdominal tenderness. Her neurologic exam is intact. She has not travelled and has no signs of an infection.

Laboratory Data: Hb 6.7 g/dL, WBC 2.4×10^9 L^{-1}, Plts 6×10^9 L^{-1}, Creatinine 0.9 mg/dL, urinalysis normal. Vitamin B12/Folate levels are normal.

LDH 645 U/L, ALP 50 U/L, AST 45 U/L, ALT 35 U/L, Total Bilirubin (Bn) 3.5 mg/dL, indirect Bn 3.0 mg/dL. ANA: 1:640 dilutions: +Anti-Sm/Ds-DNA/RNP antibodies. Complement C3/4 are both normal.

On peripheral blood smear: polychromasia and spherocytes are seen.

What is the diagnosis?

Answer 41: Subscapularis
This muscle is the strongest of the rotator cuff muscles and is the major internal rotator of the shoulder. Although less commonly torn than the supraspinatus it is often more painful as the biceps tendon is often torn at the same time. This can be managed conservatively in older patients or surgically in younger physically active individuals [1].

Answer 42: Dual energy CT scan (DECT)
If available, a DECT can provide useful information about the presence of uric acid (UA) deposition. Due to the unique chemical composition of UA there is a characteristic radiographic appearance of uric acid which is allocated a specific color and can be contrasted with calcium and soft tissue. This technique appears more sensitive in individuals with chronic disease. Radiographs are often normal in gout but in chronic gout characteristic punched out erosions can be seen in a periarticular location often with "overhanging edges" and sclerotic margins. Ultrasound and MRI are more useful in tophaceous gout [2, 3].

Answer 43: Endometriosis with history of catamenial pneumothorax
Endometrial tissue can occur outside the pelvic cavity and rarely can cause back pain and lung collapse. When patients with cyclical back pain present this diagnosis should be considered. Catamenial pneumothorax is the most common manifestation of thoracic endometriosis. The right side is involved in the majority of cases and treatment with hormonal therapy should be offered if this diagnosis is confirmed [4–6].

Answer 44
Vedolizumab is a gut specific humanized monoclonal antibody, which blocks the interaction of $\alpha_4\beta_7$ integrin with MAdCAM-1. This prevents the binding of leucocytes to gut endothelial tissue and is approved for inflammatory bowel disease (IBD). Since this drug is gut specific it has not shown efficacy in the extra intestinal manifestations of IBD. The most likely reason for the flare is lack of systemic immunosuppression following withdrawal of anti-TNF therapy. Although infusion associated side effects including arthralgia, have been described, the presence of enthesopathy and sacroiliitis makes this less likely [7].

Answer 45
Since Teriperatide has been associated with osteosarcoma in rats, prescribers are cautioned about unexplained elevations of ALP. The drug is contraindicated in patients with Paget's disease of the bone or patients at higher baseline risk for osteosarcoma. The exact association of osteosarcoma in humans taking teriperatide is unclear. Since this is a new finding the drug should be stopped and the patient should be evaluated for other causes of ALP elevation [8, 9].

Answer 46: Myasthenia gravis (MG)

This is an autoimmune disease characterized by the production of anti-acetyl choline receptor antibodies (AChR) which block the binding of ACh to the receptor. Patients present with extraocular, bulbar and proximal muscle weakness. Symptoms including diplopia are typically most pronounced at the end of the day. Twenty percent of patients present with oropharyngeal symptoms including dysphagia and dysarthria. Due to the weakness of the soft palate the patient's voice often sounds nasal. Most patients have circulating autoantibodies including to AChR, abnormal nerve conduction studies to repetitive stimulation and a positive edrophonium (Tensilon) test [10].

Answer 47: Bronchiectasis (BR)

BR is a chronic lung disease with permanent airway dilatation, mucus retention and recurrent lower respiratory tract infections. The prevalence of BR in the RA population is estimated at 2–3.1% and has been described by some as an extra-articular manifestation. Although the etiology of this association is unclear and not directly linked to smoking or the presence of autoantibodies, local colonization of the lung with bacteria may increase the risk of BR. RA-BR patients require regular follow-up, with the involvement of a multidisciplinary team, including a pulmonologist, prompt treatment of infections, and recognition of adverse effects secondary to immunosuppressive treatment [11, 12].

Answer 48: L5

The L5 nerve innervates the tibialis anterior, the foot and toe dorsiflexor, the peroneal muscles and the gluteus medius muscle.

Answer 49: Pulmonary alveolar proteinosis

Pulmonary alveolar proteinosis (PAP) is a rare disease characterized by dyspnea of gradual onset and alveolar accumulation of surfactant due to defective clearance by alveolar macrophages. It is associated with myelodysplastic syndrome, but not RA and characterized by a typical "crazy paving" pattern on CT. This pattern is caused by a combination of ground-glass opacities, septal reticulations and parenchymal consolidation. On BAL large, foamy macrophages containing eosinophilic granules are found in the endoalveolar space which stain positive for Periodic acid–Schiff (PAS) and are characteristic of PAP. The prognosis is variable and treatment involves whole lung lavage [13].

Answer 50: Evans syndrome (ES) with SLE

This patient has arthritis, serositis and antibodies consistent with SLE. She also presents with features of severe thrombocytopenia and Autoimmune Hemolytic Anemia (AIHA). ES is a rare syndrome characterized by AIHA and immune mediated thrombocytopenia (ITP) and/or immune mediated neutropenia. Since this is a diagnosis of exclusion evaluation should include measurement of serum Immunoglobulins, peripheral blood T cell subsets and possibly bone marrow biopsy (to evaluate for other etiologies such as lymphoma). Treatment initially is with high dose corticosteroids or intravenous Immunoglobulin (IVIg) [14].

References

1. Tashjian RZ. Epidemiology, natural history, and indications for treatment of rotator cuff tears. Clin Sports Med. 2012;31(4):589–604.
2. Bongartz T, Glazebrook KN, Kavros SJ, et al. Dual-energy CT for the diagnosis of gout: an accuracy and diagnostic yield study. Ann Rheum Dis. 2015;74(6):1072–7.
3. Dalbeth N, Doyle AJ. Imaging tools to measure treatment response in gout. Rheumatology (Oxford). 2018;57(Suppl 1):i27–34.
4. Z D, Fei Y, Xing X, Bo-Yin Z, Qingsan Z. Low back pain tied to spinal endometriosis. Eur Spine J. 2014;23(Suppl 2):214–7.
5. Uppal J, Sobotka S, Jenkins AL III. Cyclic sciatica and back pain responds to treatment of underlying endometriosis: case illustration. World Neurosurg. 2017;97:760.e1–3.
6. Shikino K, Ohira Y, Ikusaka M. Catamenial pneumothorax. J Gen Intern Med. 2016 Oct;31(10):1260.
7. Varkas G, Thevissen K, De Brabanter G, et al. An induction or flare of arthritis and/or sacroiliitis by vedolizumab in inflammatory bowel disease: a case series. Ann Rheum Dis. 2017;76(5):878–81. https://doi.org/10.1136/annrheumdis-2016-210233.
8. Andrews EB, Gilsenan AW, Midkiff K, et al. The US postmarketing surveillance study of adult osteosarcoma and teriparatide: study design and findings from the first 7 years. J Bone Miner Res. 2012;27(12):2429–37.
9. Miller PD. Safety of parathyroid hormone for the treatment of osteoporosis. Curr Osteoporos Rep. 2008;6(1):12–6.
10. Gilhus NE. Myasthenia gravis. N Engl J Med. 2016;375(26):2570–81.
11. Allain J, Saraux A, Guedes C, et al. Prevalence of symptomatic bronchiectasis in patients with rheumatoid arthritis. Rev Rhum Engl Ed. 1997;64(10):531–7.
12. Geri G, Dadoun S, Bui T, Del Castillo Pinol N, Paternotte S, Dougados M, et al. Risk of infections in bronchiectasis during disease-modifying treatment and biologics for rheumatic diseases. BMC Infect Dis. 2011;11:304.
13. Patel SM, Sekiguchi H, Reynolds JP, Krowka MJ. Pulmonary alveolar proteinosis. Can Respir J. 2012;19(4):243–5.
14. Domiciano DS, Shinjo SK. Autoimmune hemolytic anemia in systemic lupus erythematosus: association with thrombocytopenia. Clin Rheumatol. 2010;29(12):1427–31.

Chapter 6
Questions 51–60

© Springer International Publishing AG, part of Springer Nature 2018   71
Y. Ali, *Self Assessment in Rheumatology*,
https://doi.org/10.1007/978-3-319-89393-8_6

Question 51

A 56-year-old female presents with arthralgias and fatigue. Lab work is unremarkable apart from normocytic anemia and Howell Jolly bodies on peripheral smear. Her examination reveals a blistering rash on the elbows.

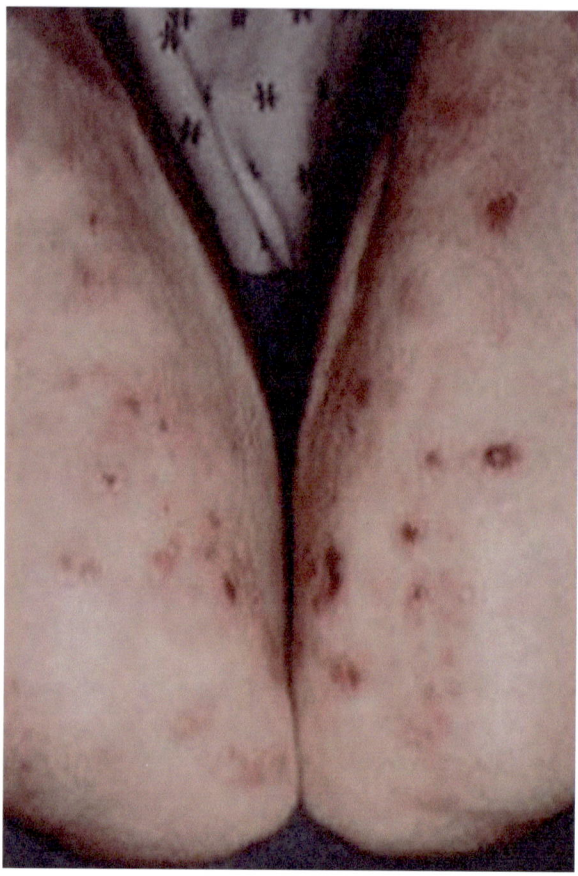

What is the most likely diagnosis?
What are the other hematologic complications of this disease?

Question 52

A 35-year-old female is referred for evaluation of + antinuclear antibodies (ANA). She is asymptomatic. Her lab work reveals ANA 1:320 homogeneous pattern; extractable nuclear antigens are negative. Hematologic and renal function values are normal and urinalysis is without sediment. Her examination is unremarkable apart from a smooth nontender goiter. The past medical history is significant for Hashimoto's thyroiditis. No rash, synovitis, or serositis is observed.

What is the most likely diagnosis?

What further treatment or investigations are warranted?

Question 53

You are asked to evaluate a 74-year-old male with joint pain. He was recently admitted after a bout of diverticulitis. On examination he has polyarticular synovitis, and arthrocentesis reveals multiple intracellular uric acid (UA) crystals diagnostic of gout. Lab values: UA = 5.5 mg/dl, WBC = 10.5, HB = 11.5, Plts = 550, and creatinine = 2.8 mg/dl.

How would you best manage this patient's gout? Why is the uric acidnormal?

Question 54

A 55-year-old female with longstanding Sjogrens syndrome (SS) presents with new onset of lethargy, hypokalemia, and nephrocalcinosis. Her metabolic profile reveals an anion gap metabolic acidosis, hypokalemia, and alkaline urine. A skeletal survey reveals diffuse osteopenia.

What complication has occurred?

Question 55

A 47-year-old patient with Crohn's disease presents for evaluation of new onset arthritis. She has a 20-year history of colitis managed with sulfasalazine and local corticosteroid suppositories. Infliximab at 5 mg/kg was recently commenced due to persistent disease activity. She arrives with new onset polyarticular joint pain. On examination she has synovitis of the small joints of the hands and a warm knee effusion. Lab work: WBC = 2.8, Hb = 11.2 g/dl, platelets = 554, ESR = 66, ANA = 1:640, RF = 54, and renal and liver studies normal.

  What is the most likely diagnosis?
  What further tests can confirm this?
  How would you manage this patient?

Question 56

A 67-year-old man presents with left groin pain. His internist has ordered a bone scan and radiograph, which he would like you to interpret. The hip radiograph reveals stage 4 osteoarthritis (OA).

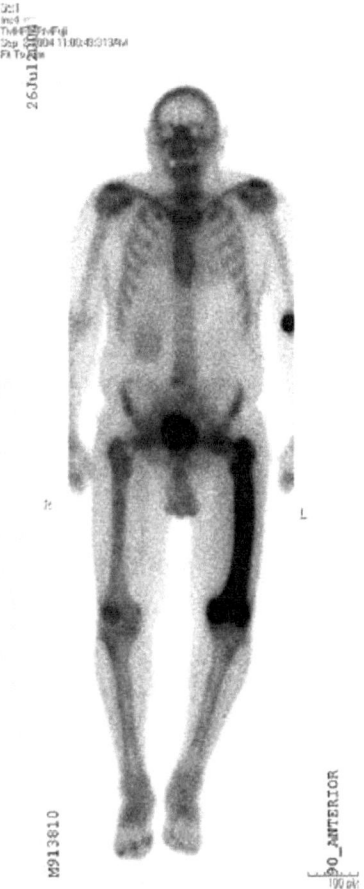

What is the most likely diagnosis?
How would you best manage this patient's bone pain?
What complications may occur?

Question 57

A 45-year-old female with 5 years of rheumatoid arthritis (RA) presents with increasing pain and stiffness. On examination she has synovitis of the metacarpo-phalangeal (mcp) and proximal interphalangeal (pip) joints with associated joint tenderness. Her current regimen includes plaquenil (hydroxychloroquine) 200 mg twice daily, sulfasalazine 3 g daily, and folate. Labs reveal ESR = 25 mm/h, + Rheumatoid Factor (RF), + Cyclic Citrullinated Peptide (CCP) antibody. CRP (C-Reactive Protein) is 162 mg/l and disease activity score (DAS) is high. Radiographs reveal periarticular erosions.

   What is the significance of the +CCP antibody?

   How would you manage her RA?

Question 58

A 68-year-old female is referred for diffuse joint pain and fatigue of 2 years duration. Her history is consistent with depression, posttraumatic stress disorder (PTSD), and hypothyroidism. Hematologic, biochemical, and immunologic studies are negative. Inflammatory markers are not elevated. On examination she has palatal hypertrophy and is markedly obese. Cardiac examination reveals a loud S2 with RV heave. Pulmonary examination is normal. She has pitting edema and multiple tender points to palpation but no synovitis.

   What is the most likely diagnosis?
   What investigations, if any, are appropriate?
   How would you manage her?

Question 59

A 74-year-old male with chronic erosive RA of 35 years duration presents with new onset bipedal edema. Current treatment regimen includes low-dose weekly Methotrexate (MTX), and 5-mg prednisone of daily. His labs reveal Hb = 10.8g/dl, MCV = 88, and platelets = 544x10^9/L. Creatinine is 0.8 mg/dl. ESR = 67 mm/h. Cardiac and pulmonary examinations are normal. An echocardiogram (ECHO) reveals increased left ventricular wall thickness, abnormal myocardial reflectivity, and a small pericardial effusion pattern.

What is the most likely diagnosis?

What further tests are warranted?

How would you manage him?

Question 60

A 25-year-old female with a 5-year history of SLE presents with increasing edema of 1-week duration. Her medications include hydroxychloroquine 200 mg twice daily. She has a history of cervical intraepithelial neoplasia and human papilloma virus (HPV). Lab data reveal Hb = 10.5g/dl, WBC = 3.2×10^9/L, and creatinine = 0.6 mg/dl. Urinalysis shows 4+ proteinuria, red cell casts, and active sediment. A renal biopsy shows active glomerulonephritis with full-house immunofluorescence interpreted as stage IV active diffuse proliferative glomerulonephritis (DPGN).

How would you manage this condition?

Answer 51: Celiac disease (CD)

This disease is more common in patients of Northern European ancestry and characterized by sensitivity to gluten. Patients present with symptoms of malabsorption, arthralgia, skin rash, and hematologic disorders. Dermatitis herpeteformis is a blistering skin rash seen in this condition. Howell Jolly bodies reflect nuclear remnants that persist due to hyposplenism. Hematologic complications of CD include anemia due to malabsorption of iron, B12, or folate; lymphoma, leucopenia, thromboembolism, and IgA deficiency [1].

Answer 52: Hashimotos thyroiditis

The ANA is most likely of no clinical significance. Up to 46% of patients with autoimmune thyroid disease have positive antinuclear antibodies. Assuming that the patient remains asymptomatic no further intervention is warranted [2].

Answer 53: Oral corticosteroids

This is a common inpatient scenario. A stable patient with renal failure is admitted and undergoes a stressful procedure that triggers gout. Treatment of acute gout involves high-dose NSAIDs, colchicine, or corticosteroids. In a patient with renal failure and diverticular inflammation, NSAIDs and colchicine should be avoided since they are poorly tolerated. A monoarticular presentation could be injected with local intraarticular corticosteroid assuming that the cultures are negative. In this patient with polyarticular gout a short burst of oral corticosteroid is the best option.

Uric acid levels fall and are often normal during an attack and should not be used as a diagnostic test [3, 4].

Answer 54: Distal type 1 renal tubular acidosis (RTA)

This is a rare but important complication of SS. Distal RTA occurs due to failure to acidify urine to a pH < 5.3. This results in anion gap acidosis, hypokalemia, nephrocalcinosis, and bone demineralization. The lymphocytes that invade the tubular epithelial cells are CD8-positive, i.e., cytotoxic T cells and similar to those found in the salivary glands of patients with Sjögren's syndrome. The same immunological process is probably operative in the renal tubulointerstitial tissue as in the salivary glands to induce the characteristic tissue changes of Sjögren's syndrome [5–7].

Answer 55: Infliximab-induced SLE

This patient presents with a new polyarticular flare after commencing infliximab. The differential diagnosis is between Crohn's related arthropathy and drug-induced SLE (DIL). The latter is more likely given the leucopenia and +ANA. Infliximab has been reported to induce antinuclear antibodies and can cause drug-induced SLE. Prompt discontinuation of the drug is warranted. Further testing includes checking antibodies to histone protein, extractable nuclear antigens, serum complements, differential cell count to look for lymphopenia, and renal function. Typically drug-induced SLE does not involve major organ systems [8].

Answer 56: Paget's disease

This bone scan shows tibial bowing and marked uptake in the left femur consistent with Paget's disease. The bone pain should be managed by oral or intravenous bisphosphonates. Zoledronic acid was approved in the USA in 2007 as a single, once annual intravenous infusion for the treatment of Paget's disease. Complications of Paget's disease include fracture, high-output heart failure, deafness, and, very rarely, osteosarcoma [9, 10].

Answer 57: The CCP antibody predicts disease severity and progression to erosions. Methotrexate should be added

She has aggressive erosive disease with elevated markers of inflammation and high-titer CCP antibody. Since she is actively symptomatic despite two disease-modifying antirheumatic drugs (DMARDs) it is time to add methotrexate(MTX). Triple therapy is superior to single agents although there are many pills to take weekly. A short bridge of corticosteroids may also be helpful in decreasing inflammatory symptoms. Some rheumatologists will argue that aggressive early use of tumor necrosis factor (TNF) antagonists or biologics is also indicated. Since these are expensive medications and the patient has not failed the "gold standard" they should be reserved unless she fails to respond to MTX. This algorithm may change as cost–benefit data on the existing agents become available and as newer, safer, and more efficacious agents are introduced [11, 12].

Answer 58: Obstructive sleep apnea with pulmonary hypertension and benign arthralgias/fibromyalgia

Patients with chronic sleep apnea develop pulmonary hypertension due to hypoxemia and develop subsequent right-sided pulmonary hypertension. A distinct relationship exists between poor sleep quality and pain intensity. This patient most likely has fibromyalgia, which is characterized by widespread pain, insomnia, and tender points. Investigations should focus around excluding an organic cause for pain, managing sleep disturbance, and treating underlying sleep apnea and depression. Physical therapy, counseling, and aerobic exercise have also been found to be useful [13].

Answer 59: This patient has developed secondary amyloidosis due to chronic inflammation

Amyloidosis is a systemic disease characterized by deposition of insoluble beta pleated sheets of protein in various organs. The diagnosis can be confirmed by congo red staining of subcutaneous fat. Although it is primary amyloidosis that usually affects the myocardium it can also occur with the secondary form. His lower extremity edema might be explained by heart failure but nephrotic syndrome also needs to be excluded. Treatment of secondary amyloidosis is often unsatisfactory and primarily involves treatment of the underlying disease [14, 15].

Answer 60: Treat with mycophenylate mofetil

This patient has class IV lupus nephritis, which, untreated, has a high risk of progression to chronic renal failure. The standard of care has been pulse dose methylprednisolone with intravenous cyclophosphamide given initially as monthly pulses and subsequently quarterly for a 2-year period. Patients with SLE who have received IV cytoxan have a higher risk of progression to cervical dysplasia, and therefore in this patient mycophenylate mofetil is a better alternative with equal efficacy and less toxicity [16–18].

References

1. Halfdanarson TR, Litzow MR, Murray JA. Hematologic manifestations of celiac disease. Blood. 2007;109(2):412–21.
2. Petri M, Karlson EW, Cooper DS, Ladenson PW. Autoantibody tests in autoimmune thyroid disease: a case-control study. J Rheumatol. 1991;18(10):1529–31.
3. Terkeltaub RA. Clinical practice. Gout N Engl J Med. 2003;349(17):1647–55.
4. Shekelle PG, Newberry SJ, FitzGerald JD, Motala A, O'Hanlon CE, Tariq A, Okunogbe A, Han D, Shanman R. Management of Gout: A Systematic Review in Support of an American College of Physicians Clinical Practice Guideline. Ann Intern Med. 2017;166(1):37–51. doi: 10.7326/M16-0461. Epub 2016.
5. Matsumura R, Kondo Y, Sugiyama T, Sueishi M, Koike T, Takabayashi K, Tomioka H, Yoshida S, Tsuchida H. Immunohistochemical identification of infiltrating mononuclear cells in tubulointerstitial nephritis associated with Sjögren's syndrome. Clin Nephrol. 1988;30(6):335–40.
6. Moutsopoulos HM, Cledes J, Skopouli FN, Elisaf M, Youinou P. Nephrocalcinosis in Sjögren's syndrome: a late sequela of renal tubular acidosis. J Intern Med. 1991;230(2):187–91.
7. Wrong OM. Immune-related potassium-losing interstitial nephritis: a comparison with distal renal tubular acidosis. QJM. 1993;86(8):513–42.
8. Watts RA. Musculoskeletal and systemic reactions to biological therapeutic agents. Curr Opin Rheumatol. 2000;12(1):49–52.
9. Bone HG. Nonmalignant complications of Paget's disease. J Bone Miner Res. 2006;21(Suppl 2):P64–8. Review
10. Keating GM, Scott LJ. Zoledronic acid: a review of its use in the treatment of Paget's disease of bone. Drugs. 2007;67(5):793–804.
11. O'Dell JR, Leff R, Paulsen G, Haire C, Mallek J, Eckhoff PJ, Fernandez A, Blakely K, Wees S, Stoner J, Hadley S, Felt J, Palmer W, Waytz P, Churchill M, Klassen L, Moore G. Treatment of rheumatoid arthritis with methotrexate and hydroxychloroquine, methotrexate and sulfasalazine, or a combination of the three medications: results of a two-year, randomized, double-blind, placebo-controlled trial. Arthritis Rheum. 2002;46(5):1164–70.
12. Curtis JR, Singh JA. The Use of Biologics in Rheumatoid Arthritis: Current and Emerging Paradigms of Care. Clinical therapeutics. 2011;33(6):679–707. doi:10.1016/j.clinthera.2011.05.044.
13. Clauw DJ. Fibromyalgia: update on mechanisms and management. J Clin Rheumatol. 2007;13(2):102–9.
14. Aresté JF, Solé JMN, Vaquero CG, García JV, Escofet DR. Secondary amyloidosis in rheumatoid arthritis. A clinical study of 29 patients. Ann Med Intern. 1999;16(12):6.
15. Voskuyl AE. The heart and cardiovascular manifestations in rheumatoid arthritis. Rheumatology. 2006;45(Suppl 4):iv4–7. Review
16. Bateman H, Yazici Y, Leff L, Peterson M, Paget SA. Increased cervical dysplasia in intravenous cyclophosphamide-treated patients with SLE: a preliminary study. Lupus. 2000;9(7):542–4.
17. Ginzler EM, Dooley MA, Aranow C, Kim MY, Buyon J, Merrill JT, Petri M, Gilkeson GS, Wallace DJ, Weisman MH, Appel GB. Mycophenolate mofetil or intravenous cyclophosphamide for lupus nephritis. N Engl J Med. 2005;353(21):2219–28.
18. Ognenovski VM, Marder W, Somers EC, Johnston CM, Farrehi JG, Selvaggi SM, McCune WJ. Increased incidence of cervical intraepithelial neoplasiain women with systemic lupus erythematosus treated with intravenous cyclophosphamide. J Rheumatol. 2004;31(9):1763–7.

Chapter 7
Questions 61–70

© Springer International Publishing AG, part of Springer Nature 2018
Y. Ali, *Self Assessment in Rheumatology*,
https://doi.org/10.1007/978-3-319-89393-8_7

Question 61

A 66-year-old male was seen with a history of recurrent oral ulceration. He has no other symptoms. PMH includes posterior uveitis and aseptic meningitis. On examination he has painful eythematous lesions on the anterior shins. Labs reveal a mild normocytic anemia.

What is the most likely diagnosis?

Question 62

A 19-year-old female with Systemic Lupus Erythematous (SLE) consults you for contraceptive advice. She is sexually active and has a history of serositis, leucopenia, and arthritis. Current medications include azathioprine 100 mg/daily and naprosyn 500 mg twice daily. Labs: WBC $= 2.4 \times 10^9$, Hb $= 10.5$g/dL, platelets $= 125 \times 10^9$/L, lupus anticoagulant present, PTT $= 55$ s, and anticardiolipin (ACA) antibody IgM/IgG strongly positive.

What advice would you give her regarding contraception?

Question 63

A 23-year-old female has new onset edema following a course of high-dose steroids for poison ivy. On examination BP = 166/110, loud S2, and clear lungs without jugular distension. She has abnormal nail fold capillary examination with dilated loops and dropout. There is no sclerodactly, malar rash, synovitis, or weakness. Urinalysis shows nephritic range proteinuria with no cellular casts. ANA is 1:10,250, normal complements, negative centromere/Scl-70/ANCA antibodies. Platelets 75×10^9/L, +schistocytes on peripheral smear.

What is the most likely diagnosis?

Question 64

A 19-year-old previously healthy student is evaluated for new onset fever, joint pain, and rash. She is sexually active but denies diarrhea, urethral discharge, or sore throat. Her symptoms occurred 1 week following her menses. There was no history of travel, tick bite, or prior joint symptoms. Physical examination reveals a febrile patient with pustular lesions over the arms and tenosynovitis of the wrist. Her immunologic and hematologic studies and renal parameters are normal. The laboratory calls to inform you of gram negative diplococci growing in the blood cultures.

What is the diagnosis and how would you treat her?

Question 65

A 77-year-old male is referred to you for the treatment of intercritical gout. His serum Uric Acid (UA) is 12.5 mg/dl and he has mild renal insufficiency with a serum creatinine of 1.6 mg/dl. Allopurinol and once daily colchicine are prescribed.

He calls your answering service 1 week later with new onset of fatigue and ecchymosis.

What complication has occurred?

Question 66

A 35-year-old female is seen for follow-up of Sjogrens syndrome due to persistent arthritis and parotitis. You consider starting azathioprine. She informs you that her sister took this medicine and had a "bad reaction with her blood."

What tests should be ordered prior to commencing this drug?

How common is this abnormality?

Question 67

A 56-year old male is seen for a second opinion. He describes several years of intermittent joint pain affecting the ankles and knees with warmth and swelling. He describes chronic weight loss and diarrhea with a prior negative colonoscopy and upper GI endoscopy. He is referred for a small bowel biopsy which reveals periodic acid-Schiff staining of specimens with inclusions within the macrophages, corresponding to bacterial structures.

What is the diagnosis?

Question 68

A 76-year-old male is referred for further management of ankylosing spondylitis. He was told he had a "bamboo spine" on routine CXR. He emphatically denies stiffness, pain, or enthesopathy. His examination shows slightly limited spine flexion, normal chest excursion, and wall-to-occiput distance of 2 in. Inflammatory markers are not elevated and he had no history of ocular disease or adolescent back pain. He declines further imaging tests.

What is the most likely diagnosis?
What other tests will facilitate the diagnosis?
What treatment is advised?

Question 69

A 73-year-old male is referred for evaluation of refractory lower extremity edema (LE). He has had slight stiffness in the proximal areas but is more concerned about his leg swelling. He denies headaches/jaw claudication or visual changes. On examination he has small joint synovitis and 3+ pitting peripheral edema. There are no signs of heart failure.

Investigations reveal normal renal function and urinalysis. Hb = 11.1 g/dl, ESR = 45 mm/h. RF/CCP antibody are negative. Ultrasound of the LE reveals no evidence of venous occlusion. A two-dimensional ECHO is normal without pericardial or right-sided dysfunction.

What is the most likely diagnosis?
What treatment is advised?
What is the prognosis?

Question 70

A 47-year-old female presents with arthralgia, rash, and parasthesias. Her examination reveals palpable purpura and peripheral neuropathy but no synovitis. She denies xerostomia, sicca symptoms, renal disease, or recurrent sinusitis. Her laboratory tests reveal modest transaminitis with low serum albumin, prolonged prothrombin time. ANA is negative but RF is moderately positive. Antineutrophil Cytoplasmic Antibody (ANCA) tests are negative.

What is the most likely diagnosis?

Answer 61: Behcet's syndrome complicated by erythema nodosum

This is a condition more commonly seen in people who live on the Silk route from the Mediterranean basin to China. There is a strong association with HLA B51. The disease is characterized by thrombophlebitis, recurrent orogenital apthous ulceration, posterior uveitis, and meningoencephalitis. Cutaneous findings include a positive pathergy test, pseudofolliculitis, or erythema nodosum. Rarely pulmonary artery aneurysms can occur [1].

Answer 62: She should be advised to use barrier protection, progesterone-only pill, or IUCDs

This patient has a prolonged partial thromboplastin time, thrombocytopenia, strongly positive ACA's, and circulating lupus anticoagulant. Although the patient has not had prior thromboses she is at high risk for developing antiphospholipid antibody syndrome in view of these blood tests. These patients are hypercoagulable and should not be given estrogen-containing products due to the increased risk of thrombosis. She should be advised to use barrier protection, progesterone-only pill, or IUCDs. The American College of Obstetricians and Gynecologists (ACOG) recommends that in SLE, estrogen-containing contraceptives be avoided in patients with vascular disease, nephritis, or ACA [2, 3].

Answer 63: Scleroderma Renal Crisis (SRC) sine scleroderma

This patient most likely has scleroderma renal crisis (SRC) sine scleroderma. Fortunately this is a rare condition but renal crisis can precede the onset of skin disease. The presence of nail bed capillary loop abnormalities, high-titer ANA, new onset renal failure, malignant hypertension, and microangiopathic hemolysis is classic for this condition. High-dose corticosteroidsare associated with SRC and should be avoided in patients with known scleroderma. Aggressive early use of angiotensin converting inhibitors (ACE) is warranted for renal protection [4, 5].

Answer 64: Disseminated gonococcal arthritis (DGI)

This patient has the classic arthritis–dermatitis syndrome characterized by tenosynovitis and purulent vesicles. DGI is more common in women, and menstruation appears to be an important risk factor. The diagnosis is established by culturing the blood, cervix, urethra, rectum, pharynx, and synovial fluid. The patient and her partner should also receive testing for chlamydia.

Treatment for DGI is an intravenous cephalosporin regimen (e.g., ceftriaxone 1 g IV every 8 h) until clinical improvement followed by an oral cephalosporin [6, 7].

Answer 65: This patient has most likely developed allopurinol-associated aplastic anemia

This condition occurs rarely and may be more common in patients with renal failure. Allopurinol should be immediately discontinued and hematologic support instituted. Although colchicine toxicity can also cause bone marrow failure this tends to occur with higher doses [8–10].

Answer 66: Thiopurine *S*-methyltransferase (TPMT) mutation
This is inherited as an autosomal dominant trait. The estimated prevalence of TPMT intermediate activity is about 10% although one in 300 people are homozygous for the gene mutation. Since TPMT activity is required to metabolize thiopurine drugs a deficiency can result in severe myelosuppression [11].

Answer 67: Whipple's disease
Whipple's disease is a rare infection caused by Tropheryma whipplei, a Gram-negative Bacillus usually found in macrophages of the lamina propria of the small intestine. The typical clinical manifestations of classic Whipple's disease are diarrhea, weight loss, malabsorption, abdominal pain, and arthralgia. Although histological detection within duodenal biopsies with "Periodic Acid Schiff" (PAS) staining still is first choice for the diagnosis, quantitative real-time PCR assay using specific oligonucleotide probes for targeting repeated sequences of Tropheryma whipplei is also available. Successful treatment can be achieved in most cases using antimicrobial therapy [12, 13].

Answer 68

1. Diffuse idiopathic hyperostosis syndrome (DISH). It is very unlikely that the patient has ankylosing spondylitis (AS). AS typically affects young men in the second and third decade of life and is characterized by stiffness of the axial skeleton and sacroiliac joints. This elderly gentleman most likely has DISH syndrome, which is a condition that involves flowing ossifications along the anterolateral aspect of four contiguous vertebra. It is of unknown etiology but usually involves the thoracic spine.
2. HLA-B27gene is present in 95% of patients with AS. A pelvic radiograph would demonstrate the absence of sacroiliac disease in DISH syndrome.
3. No treatment is indicated [14].

Answer 69: Remitting seronegative symmetrical synovitis with peripheral edema (RS3PE)
This patient has classic RS3PE with peripheral edema and symmetrical swelling but no evidence of RA. This is a rare condition that mimicks PMR and RA although there are no long-term consequences of joint damage or deformity. Patients often have modestly elevated inflammatory markers and respond well to oral corticosteroids. Prognosis is generally excellent [15].

Answer 70: Hepatitis C virus (HCV) with mixed cryoglobulinemia
This patient has evidence of chronic liver disease with decreased synthetic function. The constellation of palpable purpura, arthralgia, and neuropathy are highly suggestive of mixed cryoglubulinemia (MC). MC is quite common in HCV although only clinically apparent in about 10% of patients. It is also associated with membranoproliferative glomerulonephritis and vasculitis [16].

References

1. Sakane T, Takeno M, Suzuki N, Inaba G. Behcet's disease. N Engl J Med. 1999;341(17): 1284–91.
2. ACOG Committee on Practice Bulletins. Gynecology. ACOG practice bulletin no. 73: Use of hormonal contraception in women with coexisting medical conditions. Obstet Gynecol. 2006;107(6):1453–72.
3. Lakasing L, Khamashta M. Contraceptive practices in women with systemic lupus erythematosus and/or antiphospholipid syndrome: what advice should we be giving? J Fam Plann Reprod Health Care. 2001;27(1):7–12.
4. Steen VD. Scleroderma renal crisis. Rheum Dis Clin N Am. 1996;22:861–78.
5. Steen VD, Medsger TA Jr. Case-control study of corticosteroids and other drugs that either precipitate or protect from the development of sclerodermarenal crisis. Arthritis Rheum. 1998;41:1613–9.
6. CDC. Updated regimens, April 2007 – STD treatment guidelines. Atlanta, GA: CDC; 2006.
7. Rice PA. Gonococcal arthritis (disseminated gonococcal infection). Infect Dis Clin N Am. 2005;19(4):853–61. Review
8. Conrad ME. Fatal aplastic anemia associated with allopurinol therapy. Am J Hematol. 1986;22(1):107–8.
9. Lin YW, Okazaki S, Hamahata K, Watanabe K, Usami I, Yoshibayashi M, Akiyama Y, Kubota M. Acute pure red cell aplasia associated with allopurinol therapy. Am J Hematol. 1999;61(3):209–11.
10. Shinohara K, Okafuji K, Ayame H, Tanaka M. Aplastic anemia caused by allopurinol in renal insufficiency. Am J Hematol. 1990;35(1):68.
11. Krynetski EY, Evans WE. Genetic polymorphism of thiopurine S-methyltransferase: molecular mechanisms and clinical importance. Pharmacology. 2000;61:136–46.
12. El-Abassi R, Soliman MY, Williams F, England JD. Whipple's disease. J Neurol Sci. 2017;377:197–206.
13. Dolmans RA, Boel CH, Lacle MM, Kusters JG. Clinical manifestations, treatment, and diagnosis of tropheryma whipplei infections. Clin Microbiol Rev. 2017;30(2):529–55.
14. Atzeni F, Sarzi-Puttini P, Bevilacqua M. Calcium deposition and associated chronic diseases (atherosclerosis, diffuse idiopathic skeletal hyperostosis, and others). Rheum Dis Clin N Am. 2006;32(2):413–26. viii Review
15. Olivieri I, Salvarani C, Cantini F. RS3PE syndrome: an overview. Clin Exp Rheumatol. 2000;18(4 Suppl 20):S53–5. Review
16. Saadoun D, Landau DA, Calabrese LH, Cacoub PP. Hepatitis C-associated mixed cryoglobulinaemia: a crossroad between autoimmunity and lymphoproliferation. Rheumatology. 2007;46(8):1234–42.

Chapter 8
Questions 71–80

© Springer International Publishing AG, part of Springer Nature 2018
Y. Ali, *Self Assessment in Rheumatology*,
https://doi.org/10.1007/978-3-319-89393-8_8

Question 71

A 21-year-old patient returns from New England following a trip and is referred for arthralgia, flu-like symptoms, headache, and malaise. His examination is nonfocal apart from a fever of 100.2 °F. Laboratory data reveal Hb = 12.3 g/dl, WBC = 2.8×10^9/L, and platelets = 25×10^9/L. Wright Giemsa staining of the peripheral smear reveals morula within the neutrophils. Biochemical parameters are normal apart from a slight elevation of the LDH.

What is the most likely diagnosis?

How would you treat this?

What other conditions need to be considered?

Question 72

A 44-year-old well-nourished Caucasian female is referred for evaluation of a swollen knee. She has presented to the ER on two occasions and had the knee drained. Serial culture results are negative and no crystals have been observed. The effusions have been "bloody" although she denies trauma or anticoagulant use. She walks with a limp and is otherwise well without systemic complaints. On examination she has a swollen right knee with boggy synovial thickening and mild warmth. No other joints are involved. A knee radiograph is normal. Lab tests including ANA, RF, ESR, and lyme serology are negative. Hematologic studies are normal.

What is the most likely diagnosis?

How would you manage this patient?

What relevance is her state of nourishment?

Question 73

A 78-year-old female is referred for treatment of osteoporosis. She has a history of breast cancer in situ without skeletal involvement, and esophageal reflux. Axial T scores are −2.6, Hip −2.7.

On examination she has bilateral poor dentition and marked kyphoscoliosis. There is a history of hip and spine fracture. Calcium, vitamin D, Parathyroid Hormone (PTH), and renal function are normal. Her breast cancer is currently in remission.

Her General Practitioner (GP) has tried both residronate and alendronate, which caused GI distress.

How would you manage her osteoporosis.

What drugs should be avoided?

Question 74

A 46-year-old diabetic male has pain over the metacarpophalangeal (MCP) joints. He has about 15 min of morning stiffness. On examination he has swollen tender second/third mcp joints but no overt synovitis.

Serologies are negative and radiographs reveal hook-like osteophytes at the MCP and PIP joints.

What is the most likely diagnosis?

What tests would you order?

Question 75

A 46-year-old smoker is referred with painful shins. She has a normal examination apart from a right-sided horner's syndrome. Radiographs of the tibia and fibula are normal.

What is the next appropriate test to confirm the diagnosis?

Question 76

A 78-year-old female is seen due to a swollen right shoulder. She denies having trauma or prior history of crystal arthritis. Her shoulder examination reveals a large warm effusion with limitation of motion in all directions. A radiograph demonstrates advanced glenohumeral destruction but no calcification. Arthrocentesis reveals a bloody effusion without evidence of infection or crystals on conventional polarized microscopy; cytology is negative.

What test should you order from your laboratory that will most likely yield the diagnosis?

Question 77

A 19-year-old female with SLE presents with a new limp and right groin pain. One week prior to presentation she received high-dose intravenous corticosteroids for class IV glomerulonephritis.

On examination there are no findings apart from irritation of the right hip with rotation. A pelvic and hip radiograph are normal.

What is the most likely diagnosis? How would you manage the patient?

Question 78

A 65-year-old female is referred by the GP due to an elevated creatinine phospho-
kinase (CPK). She has a history of obstructive sleep apnea, type 2 diabetes, and
hypertension. There is no history of trauma, intramuscular injection, or dark urine.
Recently she was started on atorvastatin 20 mg daily. A routine blood test 1 month
after the lab test revealed a CPK of 525 IU/ml (nl < 250 IU/ml); no baseline level is
available. On examination, she is obese; weight 350 lb. There are no rashes, nodules, or muscle tenderness. Muscle strength is 5/5 throughout.

    What additional blood tests would you like to know?

    What management is indicated?

Question 79

A 28-year-old female patient is referred for osteoporosis. She has a 6-month history of weakness, myalgia, and 50-lb weight gain. Three months prior, she fell and fractured her pelvis. PMH is unremarkable apart from poorly controlled hypertension. Her menses are normal. She takes no medications apart from atenolol.

Lab work reveals $K = 3.2$ meq, normal renal and hematologic parameters. CPK, vitamin D, and malabsorption studies including celiac antibodies are normal. A bone DEXA scan reveals an axial T score of -3.5 and hip T score of -3.3. Corresponding Z scores are both less than -2.0.

Her examination reveals a bitemporal hemianopsia, BP 155/95, obesity, and mild muscle tenderness.

What is the most likely diagnosis?

What is the optimal treatment?

Question 80

A 32-year-old teacher presents with refractory left-sided Raynaud's and left-sided neck pain. She has no other serologic or clinical stigmata of a connective tissue disease. Treatment with calcium channel blockers, aspirin, nitrates, and alpha blockers is ineffective. Her examination reveals a diminished left radial pulse with inspiration.

Blood work is normal.

What is the most likely diagnosis?

Answer 71: Human granulocytic anaplasmosis (formerly ehrlichiosis) (HGA)
HGA is becoming a more commonly recognized cause of fever following a tick bite in the USA. The vector for this infection is the Ixodes tick, which also carries the spirochaete responsible for lyme disease(*Borrelia Burgdorferi*). Humans are affected when they impinge on small mammal/tick-infested areas. The common clinical presentation is fever, headache, and myalgia. Arthralgias, septic shock, pancytopenia, renal failure, and acute respiratory distress syndrome (ARDS) are also rare complications. Treatment is with oral doxycycline.

Coinfection with babesiosis and lyme disease can also occur and should be checked in symptomatic patients who live in endemic areas [1].

Answer 72: Pigmented villonodular synovitis(PVNS)
The differential diagnosis for a hemarthrosis includes bleeding diathesis, trauma, pseudogout, charcot joint, and PVNS. Since her hematologic indices are normal and there has been no trauma; intraarticular hemorrhage or charcot joint seem less likely. Pseudogout is typically seen in older patients with preexisting degenerative joint disease, metabolic disease, or hyperparathyroidism, and no crystals have been observed.

PVNS is a rare slow-growing benign tumor of the synovium with typical MRI findings. Treatment is arthroscopic synovectomy.

Her nourishment is relevant as scurvy can also cause recurrent hemarthrosis [2, 3].

Answer 73: Subcutaneous teriperatide would be a good choice as it is an anabolic agent that avoids the oral route
This patient is at a moderately high risk for future fracture. The most potent oral antiresorptive agents are bisphosphonates (BP), which have been shown to decrease incident vertebral and hip fractures. Unfortunately, because of her esophageal disease she is a poor candidate for BPs, which can cause GI distress. A selective estrogen modulator (SERM) such as raloxifene would be a reasonable choice given her prior breast cancer although there are no data to support a reduction in hip fracture.

Teriperatide is an anabolic agent used in patients refractory to oral agents at high risk for fracture. It is given via the subcutaneous route and generally well tolerated in patients with esophageal issues.

Intravenous bisphosphonates should be avoided in this patient given the higher incidence of osteonecrosis of the jaw (ONJ) in patients with preexisting poor dentition, malignancy, diabetes, and nicotine use [4, 5].

Answer 74: Hemochromatosis
An elevated ferritin or transferrin saturation is suggestive of hemochromatosis. Patients develop osteoarthritis of the second and third MCP joint, which may be the initial clue to the diagnosis. Iron deposition occurs in the pancreas causing diabetes. Occasionally, chondrocalcinosis is observed [6].

Answer 75: Chest X-ray
This patient most likely has a Pancoast's tumor causing hypertrophic pulmonary osteoarthropathy (HPOA). Bronchogenic carcinoma is one of the causes of HPOA and results in periostitis and clubbing. Although the cause is unknown, abnormal expression of vascular endothelial growth factor(VEGF) has been described in this condition [7].

Answer 76: Alizarin stain

This patient most likely has Milwaukee shoulder due to the presence of calcium hydroxyapatite crystals. This condition is characterized by intrarticular or periarticular hydroxyapatite crystals causing a destructive arthropathy at the glenohumeral and rotator cuff interval. The cause is unknown [8].

Answer 77: Avascular necrosis (AVN) of the femoral head

AVN results in dead trabecular bone and marrow extending to involve the subchondral plate due to local ischemia. The highest incidence of AVN of the hips occurs in patients with SLE and renal transplants, who have been exposed to high-dose steroids. Ultimately collapse of the femoral head occurs, which necessitates hip replacement. In early stage 1 AVN plain radiographs are normal and so a high level of suspicion needs to be maintained.

The patient should be evaluated by an orthopedist and avoid weight-bearing. Core decompression should be considered depending on the severity of necrosis. Since the risk of AVN is greater in patients with hypercoagulability, antiphospholipid syndrome should be excluded [9].

Answer 78: TSH, renal function

This patient has a slightly elevated CPK level without symptoms of muscle breakdown or inflammation. Given her obesity, the most likely scenario is that the CPK reflects her high muscle mass and is normal when calibrated for her BMI.

This is a common scenario in practice and in the absence of weakness, rhabdomyolysis, or pain no specific treatment is indicated. Given her cardiac risk factors she should continue the statin therapy and the CPK levels should be monitored closely.

A TSH should be checked to exclude hypothyroid myopathy. Renal function should also be checked as rhabdomyolysis is a serious complication of muscle breakdown and needs to be excluded. The absence of arthritis, Raynaud's phenomenon, or rash makes a connective tissue less likely.

Answer 79: Cushing's disease secondary to pituitary adenoma with suprasellar extension

Excessive cortisol production from an ACTH-secreting tumor results in hypertension, hypokalemia, and accelerated osteoporosis. A large mass that extends into the suprasellar fossa can place pressure on the optic chiasma resulting in visual field defects. In this case prolonged exposure of cortisol has resulted in osteoporosis. A low Z score below −2.0 raises the possibility of age inappropriate low bone mass.

The treatment of choice for classic Cushing's disease is surgical resection of the adenoma with the goal being to relieve pressure and preserve pituitary function [10].

Answer 80: Thoracic outlet syndrome due to cervical rib
This young patient has unilateral evidence of vascular insufficiency in the upper extremity. In a nonsmoker the differential diagnosis includes Raynaud's phenomenon or occlusion of the subclavian artery. Usual causes of Raynaud's phenomenon include idiopathic, hyperviscosity, atherosclerosis, connective tissue disease, or vasculitis. These are less likely in this case since the symptoms are unilateral. The patient has a positive Adson's maneuver with a diminishing pulse on inspiration suggestive of a cervical rib or fibrous band.

A CXR with apical lordotic view will show the cervical rib [11].

References

 1. Wormser GP, Dattwyler RJ, Shapiro ED, Halperin JJ, Steere AC, Klempner MS, Krause PJ, Bakken JS, Strle F, Stanek G, Bockenstedt L, Fish D, Dumler JS, Nadelman RB. Infectious Diseases Society of America practice guidelines for clinical assessment, treatment and prevention of lyme disease, human granulocytic anaplasmosis, and babesiosis. Clin Infect Dis. 2006;43(9):1089–134.
 2. Fain O. Musculoskeletal manifestations of scurvy. Joint Bone Spine. 2005;72(2):124–8.
 3. Mendenhall WM, Mendenhall CM, Reith JD, Scarborough MT, Gibbs CP, Mendenhall NP. Pigmented villonodular synovitis. Am J Clin Oncol. 2006;29(6):548–50. Review
 4. Bamias A, Kastritis E, Bamia C, et al. Osteonecrosis of the jaw in cancer treatment after bisphosphonates: incidence and risk factors. J Clin Oncol. 2005;34:8580–7.
 5. Durie BGM, Katz M, Crowley J. Osteonecrosis of the jaw and bisphosphonates. N Engl J Med. 2005;353:99–102.
 6. Jordan JM. Arthritis in hemochromatosis or iron storage disease. Curr Opin Rheumatol. 2004;16(1):62–6. Review
 7. Martinez-Lavin M. Exploring the cause of the most ancient clinical sign of medicine: finger clubbing. Semin Arthritis Rheum. 2007;36(6):380–5.
 8. Ea HK, Lioté F. Calcium pyrophosphate dihydrate and basic calcium phosphate crystal-induced arthropathies: update on pathogenesis, clinical features, and therapy. Curr Rheumatol Rep. 2004;6(3):221–7. Review
 9. Abu-Shakra M, Buskila D, Shoenfeld Y. Osteonecrosis in patients with SLE. Clin Rev Allergy Immunol. 2003;25(1):13–24. Review
10. Newell-Price J, Bertagna X, Grossman AB, Nieman LK. Cushing's syndrome. Lancet. 2006;367(9522):1605–17. Review
11. Mackinnon SE, Novak CB. Thoracic outlet syndrome. Curr Probl Surg. 2002;39(11): 1070–145. Review

Chapter 9
Questions 81–90

© Springer International Publishing AG, part of Springer Nature 2018
Y. Ali, *Self Assessment in Rheumatology*,
https://doi.org/10.1007/978-3-319-89393-8_9

Question 81

You are asked to see a 22-year-old female originally from Laos who is admitted as an inpatient. She presented with a febrile illness with quotidian spikes to 101 °F. There is associated malaise and general weakness. There has been no recent travel out of the USA for over a year and no sick contacts, tick bites, or rash. On examination she is febrile, and there is diffuse shotty lymphadenopathy, splenomegaly, and bilateral warm knee effusions. Her lab work reveals leukocytosis with lymphocytic predominance, normal renal function, mild transaminitis, and low serum albumin. Urinalysis is normal with no proteinuria or cellular activity. Microbiologic, viral, and rickettsial titers are negative. Bone marrow studies are nondiagnostic and negative for mycobacteria. CT scans of abdomen, chest, and pelvis are normal.

You order blood work: ANA +1:40, RF negative, CCP negative, ASO, Parvovirus, and urine tests for gonorrhea are negative. ESR is 115 mm/h, CRP = 372 mg/dl, and ferritin = 4500 ng/ml.

What is the most likely diagnosis?

How would you manage her?

Question 82

A 75-year-old man is referred to evaluate an elevated ESR. He has had occipital and bitemporal HA of 3-months duration with associated jaw pain and scalp tenderness. A 1-cm left temporal biopsy is negative for temporal arteritis or vasculitis. On examination he appears cachectic and has diffuse tenderness over the right temporal artery. There is lymphadenopathy and right-sided diplopia with medial rectus weakness.

Labs reveal normocytic anemia, ESR = 88 mm/h. Hepatic and renal functions are intact. Immunoelectrophoresis is without monoclonality.

What tests would you order to confirm the diagnosis?

Question 83

A 46-year-old male is admitted with new onset of rectal bleeding after having taken 1600-mg ibuprofen for an acutely swollen toe. You are asked to examine him by the colorectal surgeon for acute podagra. They are considering a colectomy to arrest the bleeding, which has failed to stop by conventional means.

On examination he has a red tender inflamed first toe with exquisite tenderness. Lab work reveals mild anemia, mild prerenal kidney dysfunction. Uric acid is normal.

How would you treat his gout?

Question 84

A 22-year-old male presents with recurrent intermittent monoarthritis affecting the toes, knees, and ankle. Arthrocentesis reveals intracellular uric acid crystals diagnostic of acute gout. Lab work: Cr = 0.6 mg/dl, UA = 14 mg/dl, CBC normal. Hepatic function is normal. Twenty-four hour urine UA is low.

What is the most likely diagnosis and cause?

Question 85

A 45-year-old female with 10 years of seropositive erosive rheumatoid arthritis presents with new onset of shortness of breath, low-grade fever, and dry cough. Her current regimen includes hydroxychloroquine 400 mg/day, prednisone 10 mg/day, sulfasalazine 3 g daily, and infliximab 5 mg/kg. She has never taken methotrexate. She resides in New England, and denies recent travel.

Examination reveals chronic rheumatoid deformities without active synovitis. Pulmonary examination reveals fine diffuse inspiratory crepitations bilaterally. A CXR describes fine perihilar reticular opacification. Blood gases revealed hypoxia, and she failed to improve with broad spectrum and empiric macrolide therapy. Lab work reveals normocytic anemia without leucocytosis. Renal, liver function and CPK are normal. LDH is markedly elevated. Peripheral smear is without hemolysis.

Bronchoscopy reveals negative stains for acid- and alcohol-fast bacilli on three occasions and PPD (TB) skin tests are negative. CMV, *Mycoplasma*, *Legionella*, Q-fever, adenovirus, influenza, *Chlamydia*, cytomegalovirus, Epstein-Barr virus, hepatitis B and C, and HIV titers are negative.

What is the most likely diagnosis?

Question 86

A 44-year-old female presents with recurrent uveitis and scleritis. She has a 3-month history of nasal discharge and shortness of breath. CXR is reported as having cavitatory lesions. Nasal mucosa is erythematous and reveals a perforation within the septum. She has no evidence of synovitis, rash, or mononeuritis on examination. Microbiologic evaluation, including TB and cocaine use is negative. PFTs reveal mild restriction and upper airway obstruction.

What is the most likely diagnosis and how would you make this diagnosis?

Question 87

A 33-year-old heterosexual monogamous firefighter is referred for bloody diarrhea and new onset of knee swelling. He is stiff for about 45 min in the morning. There is no history of travel, urethral discharge, or uveitis. On examination he has a warm left knee effusion and mild tenderness in the abdomen. Spine forward flexion is slightly limited. A painful erythematous rash is noted on the anterior shins. Lab work reveals mild microcytic anemia. ESR is 110 mm/h. Stool cultures are negative. Renal and hepatic function is preserved.

What is the most likely diagnosis and how would you confirm it? How would you initially manage his joint pain?

Question 88

A 67-year-old female with RA is referred for further management. She has multiple comorbidities including chronic renal failure, diabetes, and hypertension. She has pain in the hands, wrists, and feet with 4 h of early morning stiffness. On examination there is polyarthritis of the small joints of the hands with significant joint margin tenderness. Prednisone at 15 mg daily and weekly methotrexate (MTX) at 15 mg is commenced. You are called by the ER 1 week later where she is being seen for new onset odonophagia and dysphagia. On examination she has severe mucosal ulceration. Lab work reveals mild hyperglycemia and stable renal dysfunction.

What complication has occurred?

How could this have been prevented?

Question 89

A 68-year-old Caucasian female is referred for further management of osteoporosis. She underwent early menopause at 43 and did not receive hormone replacement. A bone density taken 2 years before revealed an axial T score of 0.5 and appendicular T score of −2.6. She was treated with calcium supplements and alendronate 70 mg weekly. Despite bisphosphonate therapy she has had several fragility fractures in the past year. A repeat DEXA is performed and this confirms a slight decline in bone mass. Serum electrolytes including alkaline phosphatase, calcium, celiac antibodies, PTH, and 25-vitamin D levels are all normal.

How would you manage this patient?

Question 90

A 41-year-old female is referred due to 4 years of recurrent sinusitis. She has failed multiple antibiotic courses and has recently developed left-sided horizontal diplopia.

Her lab work is consistent with anemia of chronic disease and an elevated ESR of 86 mm/h. Cultures for bacteria, fungi, and tubercles are negative. A CT scan of the sinuses confirms destructive pansinusitis with a nasopharyngeal mass. Serologies are consistent with a +p-ANCA, -cANCA, and -Pr3/MPO antibody. Renal and pulmonary functions are preserved.

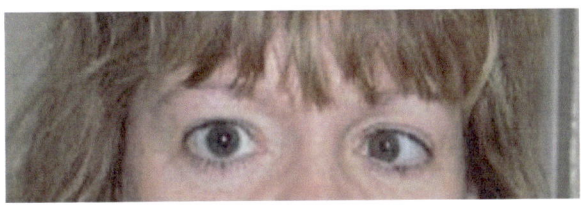

What is the differential diagnosis and most likely scenario?
What treatment is advisable?

Answer 81: The most likely diagnosis is adult onset Still's disease (AOSD)

This patient has the classic features of AOSD with spiking fever, organomegaly, derangement of liver function, leukocytosis, and a very high ferritin. This is a tricky diagnosis due to the broad differential diagnosis and potential range of infections or malignancies that can present with this type of presentation. One of the more specific clues lies in the serum ferritin, which is usually markedly elevated in AOSD and often >3000 ng/ml. The differential diagnosis of a very high ferritin (>1000 ng/ml) is limited to hemochromatosis, hemophagocytic syndrome, or AOSD.

Once infection and malignancy have been excluded treatment with high-dose steroids should be initiated in this patient who is sick with this multisystem disease. For mild flares nonsteroidal drugs may be used [1, 2].

Answer 82: Bilateral 4–6 cm TA biopsy

This elderly gentleman has symptoms that are classic for temporal arteritis (TA). Headaches and jaw claudication in the setting of a markedly elevated ESR should raise suspicion for TA. Unfortunately this is a disease of discontinuity and characterized by skip lesions on TA biopsy. Ideally a 4- to 6-cm biopsy should be obtained and a bilateral biopsy will increase the sensitivity, albeit marginally. In this case the 1-cm biopsy length is inadequate.

TA responds to high-dose prednisone and untreated can cause optic arteritis resulting in blindness. Opthalmoplegia has also been described. Myasthenia gravis or a space-occupying lesion would not cause bilateral headaches, jaw claudication, or scalp tenderness. If the clinical suspicion is high and an inadequate biopsy is obtained it should be repeated. Another option would be to obtain a color duplex ultrasound, which, in the right hands, can reveal a "halo" sign that is suggestive of active arteritis [3–7].

Answer 83: Intraarticular (IA) corticosteroid injection

This patient has acute podagra in the setting of an acute NSAID-induced gastrointestinal bleed. An IA injection of steroid is the optimal management in this patient. Colchicine is contraindicated given the renal impairment and potential to further irritate the GI tract [8].

Answer 84: Congenital under excretion of uric acid (UA) due to a tubular defect

The majority of people with gout are congenital under excretors of UA. The exact mechanism has not been elucidated but it is related to decreased secretion, increased reabsorption, or decreased filtration of UA. Overproduction of UA occurs in less than 10% of patients. Lesch Nyhan syndrome secondary to hypoxanthine guanine phosphoribosyl transferase deficiency (HGPRT) would cause an overproduction of UA and increased 24-h urinary uric acid excretion [9, 10].

Answer 85: Pneumocystis jiroveci (carinii) pneumonia (PCP)

This patient who is receiving anti-TNF therapy presents with an acute pulmonary decompensation characterized by dyspnea, hypoxemia, and an elevated LDH level. Since she is significantly immunosuppressed, an opportunistic infection is the most likely scenario. Rheumatoid lung disease, bronchiolitis obliterans with organizing pneumonia (BOOP) are also in the differential diagnosis. RA-associated lung disease tends to present more insidiously with pleural involvement and is usually not associated with elevated LDH levels.

PCP is caused by a unicellular eukaryote and is a rare cause of infection in immunocompetent individuals. The diagnostic gold standard is a broncheoalveolar lavage (BAL) with cytologic confirmation of induced sputum samples. LDH levels are a sensitive but poorly specific indicator of PCP. Since this infection is associated with high mortality a high index of suspicion is required [11–13].

Answer 86: Wegener's granulomatosis (WG)

This patient presents with recurrent sinusitis, inflammatory eye disease, and cavitatory lung lesions typical for WG. The definitive diagnosis is made by confirming the presence of noncaseating granulomas on biopsy. Serological tests include the presence of antineutrophil cytoplasmic antibodies (c-ANCA), which have a sensitivity of about 60–88%. Antibodies to proteinase 3 (PR-3) are highly sensitive in active WG (90%). Other features of WG include subglottic stenosis, pauciimmune glomerulonephritis, mononeuritis multiplex, and arthritis. In this patient other causes of cavitatory lung lesions such as infection need to be excluded prior to treatment [14, 15].

Answer 87: Inflammatory bowel disease-related arthropathy

This gentleman presents with a syndrome of bloody diarrhea, erythema nodosum, and oligoarthritis. This pattern is most classic for inflammatory bowel disease (IBD). Ideally his knee should be drained and fluid sent to confirm a sterile effusion. Colonoscopy with biopsy will confirm the diagnosis of IBD.

Initial treatment of his joint disease can involve local intraarticular injections, analgesic medications, and judicious use of anti-inflammatory medications with close collaboration with the gastroenterologist. Axial spondylitis may respond to physical therapy. The response to DMARD therapy for peripheral and axial arthritis is often disappointing. Monoclonal antibody therapy including anti IL12/23 (Ustekinumab) and anti-TNF agents (infliximab and adalimumab), in contrast, work well in this situation [16, 17, 18].

Answer 88: MTX mucositis

This patient with renal failure has developed mucositis from the methotrexate (MTX). Mucosal toxicity is a well-known complication of MTX and predisposing factors include folate deficiency, renal failure, and hypoalbuminemia. There are also various genetic polymorphisms that may predict toxicity and response to MTX. The dose of MTX should be adjusted in patients with renal failure.

This complication may have been prevented by the use of a lower dose and prophylactic daily folic acid [19, 20].

Answer 89: The optimal choice for this patient is an anabolic agent such as teriperatide or abaloperatide

This patient has multiple risk factors for osteoporosis including early menopause, sex, race, and prior fracture. Assuming that she is compliant then the fact that she is fracturing despite bisphosphonate (BP) therapy indicates that she is a true BP failure.

Teriperatide has an alternative mechanism of action to BP and stimulates osteoblasts as opposed to inhibiting osteoclasts. Osteoporosis experts have developed a consensus opinion, published in the spring of 2004, to help clinicians identify appropriate patients for teriperatide therapy. Indications for its use were as follows: (1) history of vertebral fracture, T score of −3.0 or below, or age greater than 69 years, (2) fracture or unexplained bone loss in patients on antiresorptive therapy, and (3) intolerance of oral bisphosphonate therapy. Contraindications for teriperatide therapy listed include hypercalcemia, Paget's disease, a history of irradiation to the skeleton, sarcoma, or malignancy involving bone [21].

Answer 90: Wegener's granulomatosis (WG)

This 41-year-old patient presents with a 4-year history of recurrent sinusitis in the setting of a positive P-ANCA, destructive nasopharyngeal mass, and ophthalmoplegia.

The differential diagnosis includes infection with a refractory organism, such as mucormycosis or tuberculosis, malignancy, midline granuloma, or vasculitis. Infection and malignancy seem less likely given the chronicity and lack of positive cultures.

Although most patients with WG have antibodies to proteinase-3 and positive c-ANCA antibodies, a small minority have antibodies to p-ANCA.

This patient's inflammation has extended into the sinuses and cavernous sinus causing cranial neuropathy and ophthalmoplegia.

Optimal treatment involves oral corticosteroids and oral daily cyclophosphamide. Prior to the introduction of cytotoxic drugs this was a disease of very high mortality [14, 22, 23].

References

1. Efthimiou P, Georgy S. Pathogenesis and management of adult-onset Still's disease. Semin Arthritis Rheum. 2006;36(3):144–52.
2. Zandman-Goddard G, Shoenfeld Y. Ferritin in autoimmune diseases. Autoimmun Rev. 2007;6(7):457–63.
3. Butteriss DJ, Clarke L, Dayan M, Birchall D. Use of colour duplex ultrasound to diagnose giant cell arteritis in a case of visual loss of uncertain aetiology. Br J Radiol. 2004;77(919):607–9.
4. Lazaridis C, Torabi A, Cannon S. Bilateral third nerve palsy and temporal arteritis. Arch Neurol. 2005;62(11):1766–8. Review

5. Pless M, Rizzo JF III, Lamkin JC, Lessell S. Concordance of bilateral temporal artery biopsy in giant cell arteritis. J Neuroophthalmol. 2000;20(3):216–8.
6. Salvarani C, Cantini F, Boiardi L, Hunder GG. Polymyalgia rheumatica and giant-cell arteritis. N Engl J Med. 2002;347(4):261–71. Review
7. Seo P, Stone JH. Large-vessel vasculitis. Arthritis Rheum. 2004;51(1):128–39. Review
8. Keith MP, Gilliland WR. Updates in the management of gout. Am J Med. 2007;120(3):221–4. Review
9. Emmerson BT, Nagel SL, Duffy DL, Martin NG. Genetic control of the renal clearance of urate: a study of twins. Ann Rheum Dis. 1992;51:375.
10. Lesch M, Nyhan WL. A familial disorder of uric acidmetabolism and central nervous system function. Am J Med. 1964;36:561.
11. Butt AA, Michaels S, Kissinger P. The association of serum lactate dehydrogenase level with selected opportunistic infections and HIV progression. Int J Infect Dis. 2002;6(3):178–81.
12. Kaur N, Mahl TC. Pneumocystisjiroveci (carinii) pneumonia after infliximab therapy: a review of 84 cases. Dig Dis Sci. 2007;52(6):1481–4.
13. Mutlu GM, Mutlu EA, Bellmeyer A, Rubinstein I. Pulmonary adverse events of anti-tumor necrosis factor-alpha antibody therapy. Am J Med. 2006;119(8):639–46. Review
14. Bosch X, Guilabert A, Font J. Antineutrophil cytoplasmic antibodies. Lancet. 2006;368(9533):404–18. Review
15. Seo P, Stone JH. The antineutrophil cytoplasmic antibody-associated vasculitides. Am J Med. 2004;117(1):39–50. Review
16. Padovan M, Castellino G, Govoni M, Trotta F. The treatment of the rheumatological manifestations of the inflammatory bowel diseases. Rheumatol Int. 2006;26(11):953–8. Review
17. Van den Bosch F, Kruithof E, De Vos M, De Keyser F, Mielants H. Crohn's disease associated with spondyloarthropathy: effect of TNF-alpha blockade with infliximab on articular symptoms. Lancet. 2000;356(9244):1821–2.
18. Peluso R, Manguso F, Vitiello M, Iervolino S, Di Minno MND. Management of arthropathy in inflammatory bowel diseases. Therapeutic Advances in Chronic Disease. 2015;6(2):65-77. doi:10.1177/2040622314563929.
19. Grosflam J, Weinblatt ME. Methotrexate: mechanism of action, pharmacokinetics, clinical indications, and toxicity. Curr Opin Rheumatol. 1991;3(3):363–8. Review
20. Takatori R, Takahashi KA, Tokunaga D, Hojo T, Fujioka M, Asano T, Hirata T, Kawahito Y, Satomi Y, Nishino H, Tanaka T, Hirota Y, Kubo T. ABCB1 C3435T polymorphism influences methotrexate sensitivity in rheumatoid arthritis patients. Clin Exp Rheumatol. 2006;24(5):546–54.
21. Miller PD, Bilezikian JP, Deal C, et al. Clinical use of teriperatide in the real world: initial insights. Endocr Pract. 2004;10:139.
22. Erickson VR, Hwang PII. Wegener's granulomatosis: current trends in diagnosis and management. Curr Opin Otolaryngol Head Neck Surg. 2007;15(3):170–6. Review
23. Foster WP, Greene JS, Millman B. Wegener's granulomatosis presenting as ophthalmoplegia and optic neuropathy. Otolaryngol Head Neck Surg. 1995;112(6):758–62.

Chapter 10
Questions 91–100

© Springer International Publishing AG, part of Springer Nature 2018
Y. Ali, *Self Assessment in Rheumatology*,
https://doi.org/10.1007/978-3-319-89393-8_10

Question 91

A 67-year-old diabetic African American male is referred for evaluation of chronic right ankle pain. There is a distant history of trauma and poorly controlled diabetes. He denies podagra, and serum uric acid is normal. On examination he has fair peripheral circulation, pes planus with mild ankle tenderness at the tibiotalar joint, and glove and stocking neuropathy is present. His radiograph shows diffuse demineralization and Lisfranc dislocation of the midtarsus. The joint is tapped and hemarthrosis is noted.

 What is the most likely diagnosis?

 Who was Lisfranc?

Question 92

A 58-year-old female from the Dominican Republic with seropositive RA of 20-year duration is seen due to fever, dyspnea, and malaise. She commenced anti-TNF therapy 1 month prior to her presentation due to poorly controlled RA. Her current medications include methotrexate, folate, celecoxib, and infliximab. Her examination shows a low-grade temperature of 100.5 °F. She has chronic synovitis of the mcp/pip and wrist joints with bibasilar end inspiratory crepitations on pulmonary examination. Serum and urine microbiologic studies are negative. A CXR reveals chronic bibasilar fibrosis and a new apical infiltrate.

What is the major clinical concern in this patient?

Question 93

You are asked to see a 46-year-old alcoholic male to help with the management of presumed gout. He presented with acute bilateral ankle pain and swelling. He has chronic low back stiffness. The admitting physician has performed arthrocentesis of the ankle joint, which confirmed type 2 inflammatory fluid without crystals. Lab work reveals intact hematologic and renal function and UA = 8.4 mg/dl.

On examination he has bilateral tenderness over the right metatarsal heads, thickening of the Achilles tendon with exquisite tenderness, and warm bilateral ankle effusions. Radiographs of the spine confirm right sacroiliac fusion. He is treated with colchicine without any improvement.

What is the most likely diagnosis?

What else would you look for on examination?

Question 94

A 27-year-old female with SLE is referred with new onset pleuritic chest pain. She has a history of arthritis and mucositis, which has been controlled on NSAIDs and antimalarial agents. She has a history of two second trimester miscarriages.

On examination she has sinus tachycardia, RV heave, and a loud P2. Diffuse livedo reticularis is noted. Lung examination is clear and CXR appears normal apart from slightly oligemic fields. She is mildly hypoxic and is using accessory muscles of respiration.

What is the most likely diagnosis?

Question 95

A 78-year-old female is admitted with malaise, fever to 101 °F and unintentional weight loss. She has a 45-year history of seropositive erosive RA controlled on methotrexate and more recently intravenous anti-TNF therapy. She has known interstitial lung disease. On examination she is cachectic, with chronic deformities and low-grade synovitis. Her lung examination reveals coarse bibasilar crepitations. She has axillary lymphadenopathy and bipedal edema. Lab work reveals a normocytic anemia, mild eosinophilia, and hypoalbuminemia but otherwise intact renal and hepatic function. Urinalysis is benign.

Viral, rickettsial, and microbiologic studies are normal; a CT scan reveals marked hilar lymphadenopathy and chronic fibrotic changes at the lung bases. A tuberculin skin test is negative.

What is the most likely diagnosis?

Question 96

A 46-year-old male immigrant is admitted for further evaluation of a pulmonary artery aneurysm noted on an incidental CXR. He has a prior history of uveitis and arthritis. On examination there is hypophyon, erythema nodosum, and oral ulceration.

What is the most likely diagnosis?

Question 97

A 67-year-old African American female with dialysis-dependent renal failure is evaluated for recurrent carpal tunnel syndrome. She has had two injections in the past 6 months, which were of temporary benefit. On examination she has atrophy of the thenar eminens and weakness of opponens muscles. Phalen's sign is positive and her grip is diminished.

What complication has occurred?

Question 98

A middle-aged Han Chinese male presents with chronic tophaceous gout. He is placed on allopurinol and develops acute Stevens-Johnson syndrome (SJS).

Could this have been avoided?

Question 99

You are asked to see a patient with refractory erythema nodosum. He is a 46-year-old ex-intravenous drug abuser who has had painful raised lesions over his shins for 4 months. He also complains of low-grade fever, arthralgia, and abdominal pain. He has lost 15 lbs in 6 months. On examination temperature is 38.3 °C, and there is evidence of clubbing and tender raised nodules over the anterior shins. His cardiac examination reveals a 3/6 ejection systolic murmur at the right sternal border and 2/6 early diastolic murmur. BP = 166/64. Pulmonary examination is normal, and abdominal examination reveals tenderness in the RUQ. A CXR is normal.

What diagnostic test should be performed?

Question 100

A 29-year-old female medical resident is seen for refractory foot pain of 1-week duration. Her past medical history is significant for anorexia nervosa for which she attends monthly counseling classes. Her weight is 87 lbs., height 5′6″. On examination she has diffuse tenderness at the midfoot. She denies trauma or swelling.

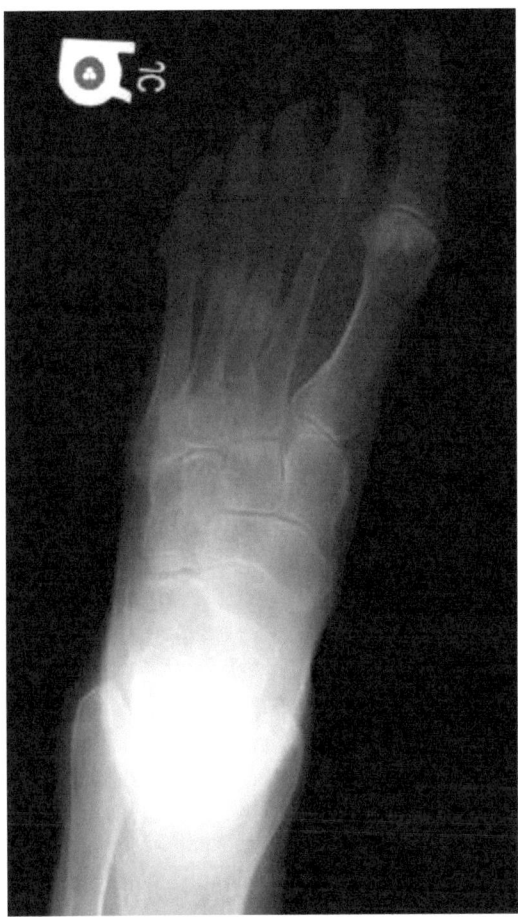

What is the diagnosis?

Answer 91: Charcot joint

This patient has a classic Charcot joint, which is characterized by damage secondary to loss of sensation that occurs due to the patient's underlying diabetes. The features of a Charcot joint include fragmentation of bone, progressive destruction, and disorganization. Although there are many causes, diabetic neuropathy is the commonest cause in the western world. Lisfranc dislocation implies disruption of the joint between the rigid midfoot and more supple weight-bearing forefoot. Arthrocentesis frequently yields a hemarthrosis.

Lisfranc was Napolean's surgeon who described a technique to amputate the forefoot in soldiers suffering from frostbite [1].

Answer 92: Tuberculosis (TB)

This patient has developed a new apical infiltrate in the setting of anti-TNF therapy. TNF is a pleiotropic molecule important in immune surveillance and host defense. It is also important in granuloma formation and maintenance. TNF-deficient knock-out mice develop fatal TB and listeriosis. Reactivation of TB is a well-recognized complication of anti-TNF therapy, and patients should be screened with skin testing prior to initiation of therapy [2–4].

Answer 93: Ankylosing spondylitis (AS)

This 46-year-old male presents with axial stiffness, metatarsal inflammation, enthesopathy, and sacroiliitis. This is highly suggestive of a reactive arthritis or AS. Gout has been effectively excluded by the absence of urate crystals and would not typically present with Achilles tendonitis or sacroiliitis.

Other things to examine for would be digital pitting, psoriatic plaques, stigmata of inflammatory bowel disease, urogenital infection, or uveitis. The elevated uric acid is of no clinical significance and the colchicine should be stopped [5].

Answer 94: Pulmonary embolus

This patient with SLE most likely has antiphospholipid syndrome (APS) with a history of recurrent pregnancy loss and livedo reticularis. Her examination reveals elevated right-sided pulmonary pressure consistent with right ventricular strain. Pericarditis should also be considered although it would be less likely given the physical findings. APS is a disease of recurrent vascular thrombosis and/or fetal loss associated with antibodies to membrane phospholipids. Approximately 40% of patients with SLE have anticardiolipin antibodies but only 10% have APS syndrome [6].

Answer 95: Lymphoma

This patient with chronic RA presents with fever, lymphadenopathy, eosinophilia, and weight loss in the setting of a negative infectious disease evaluation. The differential diagnosis includes infection, TB, and lymphoma. The latter diagnosis is most likely given the negative microbiologic studies.

Patients with chronic RA are predisposed to lymphoma, and although not clear, in 2018 this risk might be further amplified by concomitant anti-TNF therapy in certain groups of individuals. Patients with the most severe disease activity scores have the greatest risk of developing lymphomas.

When using biologic agents the benefits of treatment must be weighed against potential toxicity [7, 8, 9].

Answer 96: Behcet's syndrome

This patient has classic Behcet's syndrome (BS), which is an HLA-B51-associated disease characterized by recurrent orogenital ulceration, thrombophlebitis, uveitis, and vasculitis. Skin lesions include erythema nodosum, abnormal pathergy, and folliculitis.

The etiology is unknown but this is a disease with racial preference along the old Silk route from the Mediterranean to China. Pulmonary artery aneurysms are a rare cause of pulmonary hemorrhage and should raise the suspicion of BS [10–12].

Answer 97: B2 amyloid

Dialysis-related amyloidosis (DRA) is a complication of end-stage renal disease that results from retention of beta2-microglobulin (beta2M) and its deposition as amyloid fibrils into osteoarticular tissue. The clinical manifestations usually develop after several years of dialysis dependence and include carpal tunnel syndrome, destructive arthropathy, bone cysts, and fractures. Risk factors for the development of DRA include age, duration of dialysis treatment, use of low-flux dialysis membrane, use of low-purity dialysate, monocyte chemoattractant protein-1 GG genotype, and apolipoprotein E4 allele. This has become less common after the introduction of a high flux hemodialysis membrane.

Surgical management is usually successful but can result in recurrence. An extended release procedure may be more successful [13, 14].

Answer 98

HLA-B*5801 allele has been associated with allopurinol-induced severe cutaneous adverse reactions and this appears more common in certain racial subgroups such as Han Chinese, Korean or those of Thai descent. Although the risk of SJS is only between 0.1% and 0.4%, genetic testing is recommended in these racial groups prior to starting allopurinol. Starting a lower dose of allopurinol has also been shown to result in a fewer cases of drug induced hypersensitivity [15–17].

Answer 99: Blood cultures

This patient has endocarditis with valvular insufficiency and probable streptococcal bacteremia. Streptococcus is a common cause of erythema nodosum (EN). Other causes include sarcoidosis, TB, yersinia, fungal infections, inflammatory bowel disease, Behcet's disease, and drugs such as sulfonamides [18, 19].

Answer 100: Metatarsal fracture

Because of anorexia nervosa and low body mass, this patient is at a higher risk for osteoporosis and fragility fracture. This radiograph clearly shows two healing metatarsal fractures, which are the cause of the patient's pain. The decreased bone density in patients with anorexia nervosa (AN) is due to the many effects on bone metabolism of amenorrhea, reduced levels of insulin-like growth factor-1 (IGF-1), high cortisol levels, and weight loss. Although bisphosphonateshave been used, the most effective treatment involves resumption of menses and weight restoration [20, 21].

References

1. Tomas MB, Patel M, Marwin SE, Palestro CJ. The diabetic foot. Br J Radiol. 2000;73(868):443–50. Review
2. Crum NF, Lederman ER, Wallace MR. Infections associated with tumor necrosis factor-alpha antagonists. Medicine. 2005;84(5):291–302. Review
3. Flynn JL, Goldstein MM, Chan J, Triebold KJ, Pfeffer K, Lowenstein CJ, Schreiber R, Mak TW, Bloom BR. Tumor necrosis factor-α is required in the protective immune response against *Mycobacterium tuberculosis* in mice. Immunity. 1995;2:561–72.
4. Hamilton CD. Tuberculosis in the cytokine era: what rheumatologists need to know. Arthritis Rheum. 2003;48(8):2085–91. Review
5. Reveille JD, Arnett FC. Spondyloarthritis: update on pathogenesis and management. Am J Med. 2005;118(6):592–603. Review
6. Lockshin MD. Update on antiphospholipid syndrome. Bull NYU Hosp Jt Dis. 2006;64(1–2):57–9.
7. Franklin J, Lunt M, Bunn D, Symmons D, Silman A. Incidence of lymphoma in a large primary care derived cohort of cases of inflammatory polyarthritis. Ann Rheum Dis. 2006;65:617–22.
8. Wolfe F, Michaud K. Lymphoma in rheumatoid arthritis: the effect of methotrexate and anti-tumor necrosis factor therapy in 18,572 patients. Arthritis Rheum. 2004;50(6):1740–51.
9. Mercer LK, Galloway JB, Lunt M, et al. Risk of lymphoma in patients exposed to antitumour necrosis factor therapy: results from the British Society for Rheumatology Biologics Register for Rheumatoid Arthritis Annals of the Rheumatic Diseases. Published Online First: 08 August 2016. doi: 10.1136/annrheumdis-2016-209389.
10. Alpagut U, Ugurlucan M, Dayioglu E. Major arterial involvement and review of Behcet's disease. Ann Vasc Surg. 2007;21(2):232–9. Review
11. Uzun O, Akpolat T, Erkan L. Pulmonary vasculitis in Behcet disease: a cumulative analysis. Chest. 2005;127(6):2243–53. Review
12. Yazici H, Fresko I, Yurdakul S. Behçet's syndrome: disease manifestations, management, and advances in treatment. Nat Clin Pract Rheumatol. 2007;3(3):148–55. Review
13. Dember LM, Jaber BL. Dialysis-related amyloidosis: late finding or hidden epidemic? Semin Dial. 2006;19(2):105–9. Review
14. Wilson SW, Pollard RE, Lees VC. Management of carpal tunnel syndrome in renal dialysis patients using an extended carpal tunnel release procedure. J Plast Reconstr Aesthet Surg. 2008;61(9):1090–4.
15. Jutkowitz E, Dubreuil M, Lu N, et al. The cost-effectiveness of HLA-B*5801 screening to guide initial urate-lowering therapy for gout in the United States. Semin Arthritis Rheum. 2017;46(5):594–600.
16. Saito Y, Stamp LK, Caudle KE, Hershfield MS, et al. Clinical pharmacogenetics implementation consortium (CPIC) guidelines for human leukocyte antigen B (HLA-B) genotype and allopurinol dosing: 2015 update. Clin Pharmacol Ther. 2015;99(1):36–7.
17. Stamp LK, Taylor WJ, Jones PB, Dockerty JL, et al. Starting dose is a risk factor for allopurinol hypersensitivity syndrome: a proposed safe starting dose of allopurinol. Arthritis Rheum. 2012;64(8):2529–36.
18. Mert A, Kumbasar H, Ozaras R, Erten S, Tasli L, Tabak F, Ozturk R. Erythema nodosum: an evaluation of 100 cases. Clin Exp Rheumatol. 2007;25(4):563–70.
19. Mert A, Ozaras R, Tabak F, Pekmezci S, Demirkesen C, Ozturk R. Erythema nodosum: an experience of 10 years. Scand J Infect Dis. 2004;36(6–7):424–7.
20. Do Carmo I, Mascarenhas M, Macedo A, Silva A, Santos I, Bouça D, Myatt J, Sampaio D. A study of bone density change in patients with anorexia nervosa. Eur Eat Disord Rev. 2007;15(6):457–62.
21. Wolfert A, Mehler PS. Osteoporosis: prevention and treatment in anorexia nervosa. Eat Weight Disord. 2002;7(2):72–81. Review

Chapter 11
Questions 101–110

© Springer International Publishing AG, part of Springer Nature 2018
Y. Ali, *Self Assessment in Rheumatology*,
https://doi.org/10.1007/978-3-319-89393-8_11

Question 101

A 59-year-old diabetic male has pain over the anterior hip and groin. He has recently had angina and has started a vigorous exercise regimen. On examination there is clicking of the hip with flexion but no pain with rotation. Distal neurovascular examination is intact. A radiograph of the right hip and pelvis is normal.

What is the most likely diagnosis?

How would you treat him?

Question 102

A 35-year-old markedly obese female is referred for evaluation of scleroderma. She is asymptomatic but has limited sclerodactly and skin thickening of the face, digits. Nailfold examination shows dilated capillary loops. Lab and urine data are normal. She is diagnosed with CREST syndrome on the basis of esophageal dysfunction and Raynauds.

Cardiac examination reveals a normal S2, and pulmonary examination is clear without rales.

A baseline 2D ECHO reveals a PA pressure of 45 mmHg (nl < 25) but PFTs and DLCO are normal.

What is the next appropriate step?

Question 103

A 28-year-old female with SLE is diagnosed with class 4 nephritis. She is started on immunosuppressive therapy with pulse cyclophosphamide, prednisone, and furosemide.

Three months after the initial presentation she is admitted with hypertension and has a witnessed tonic clonic seizure in the ER. Her BP is 190/115 and she appears post ictal when you examine her. There is no rash, synovitis, or evidence of serositis. An LP is unremarkable without evidence for infection or cerebritis.

A brain MRI reveals multiple hyperintensity lesions in the occipital lobe.

What complication has occurred?

Question 104
A 25-year-old female has had low back pain for 6 months. She has an unremarkable
past history apart from one prior episode of uveitis. Review of systems is negative
for diarrhea, urethral discharge/travel, or constitutional symptoms. Her examination
reveals a positive FABER sign and tenderness over the lower lumbosacral spine and
sacroiliac joint.

The rest of the joint and skin examination is normal apart from subungual hyperkeratosis and oil spots.

What is the most likely diagnosis?

Question 105

A 67-year-old Caucasian female is referred for left forearm pain for 2 months duration. She describes pain that only occurs with activity. Her PMH includes newly
diagnosed PMR, CAD, and spinal stenosis. Her current medications include prednisone 5 mg daily, aspirin, and atenolol. On examination she is mildly cushingoid
with an absent left radial pulse. There is no peripheral synovitis, and examination of
the forearm and elbow joint is unremarkable. Resisted extension of the wrist fails to
reproduce the pain. There is a faint left subclavian bruit.

Her laboratory data reveal an elevated ESR of 80 mm/h, and normal renal and
biochemical parameters. She has a mild normocytic anemia.

What is the most likely scenario?

What is the next best step to evaluate this?

Question 106

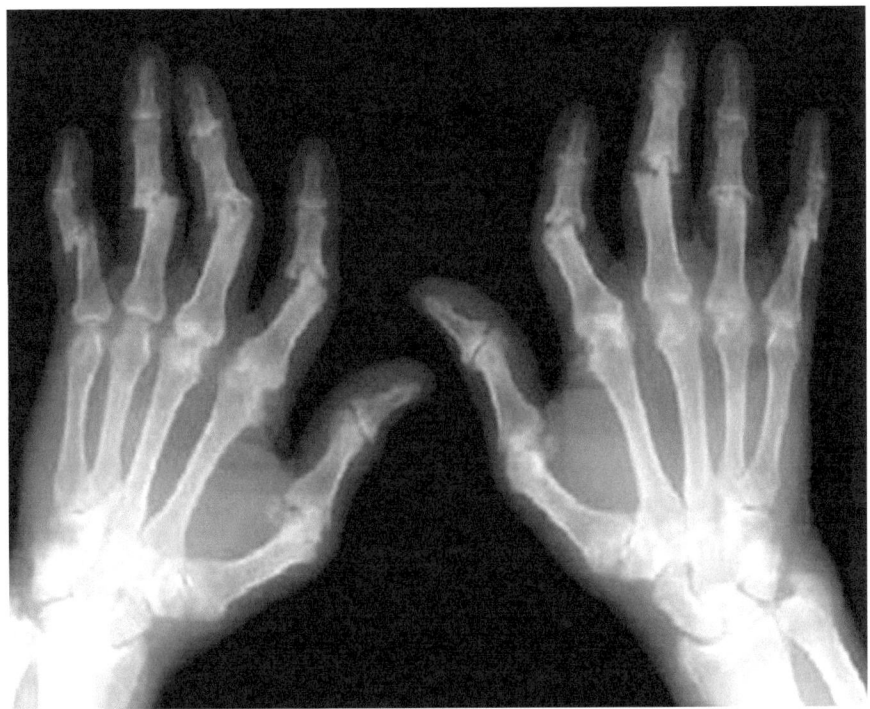

What is the diagnosis?

Question 107

This patient has severe hip pain.

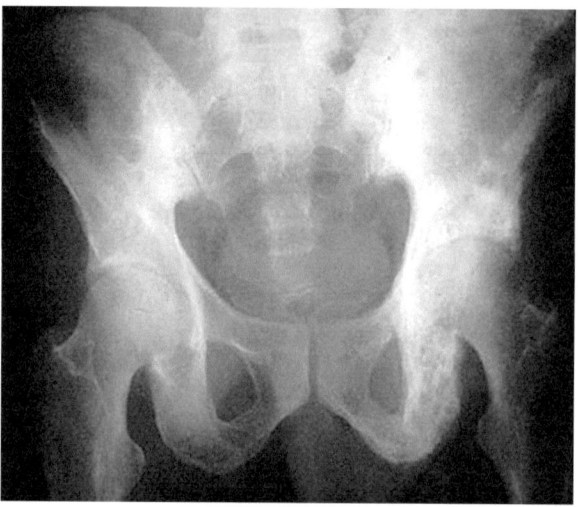

What does the X-ray show and what advice would you give to the orthopaedic surgeon?

Question 108

This patient has postpartum pain.

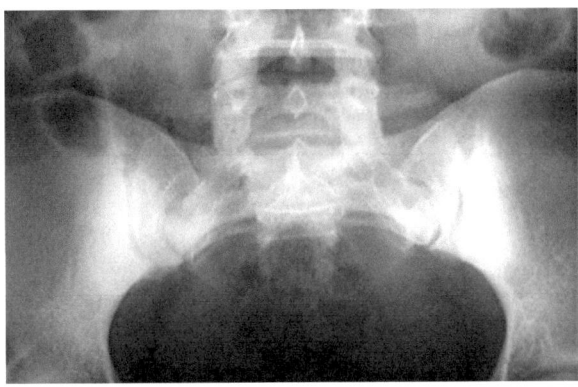

What does the X-ray show?

Question 109

This patient has refractory wrist pain.

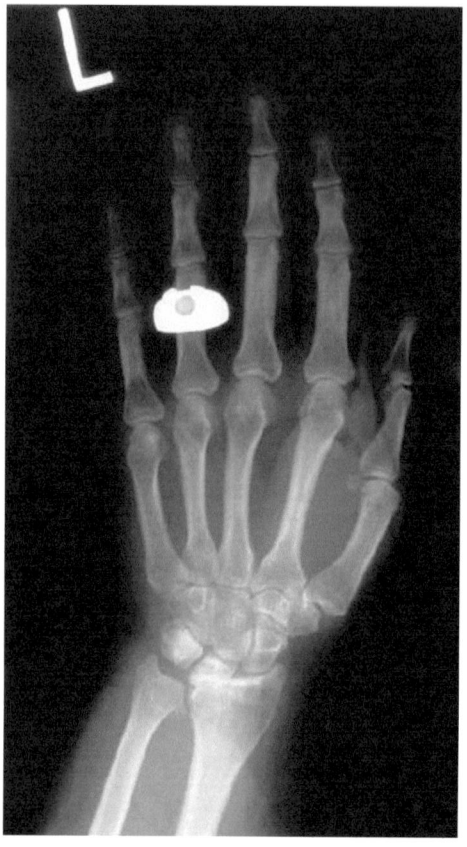

What is the diagnosis and what does the radiograph show?

Question 110
A 60-year male is evaluated with a history of spinal cord injury and knee pain.

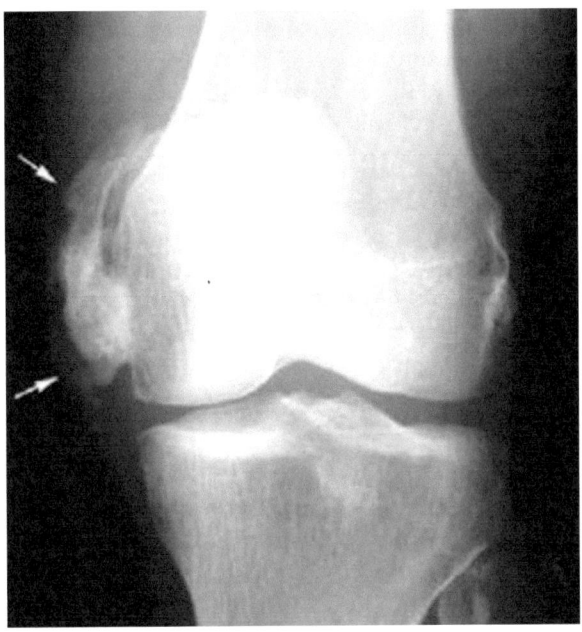

What does the X-ray show?

Answer 101: Iliopsoas bursitis

The iliopsoas muscle passes anterior to the pelvic brim and hip capsule in a groove between the anterior inferior iliac spine laterally and iliopectineal eminence medially. It acts as one of the hip flexors and is occasionally injured in excessive hip flexion or trauma. Patients often have an insidious onset of anterior thigh pain, which often radiates down to the knee and is associated with hip clicking.

Treatment involves physical therapy to alleviate pain, spasm, and swelling [1].

Answer 102: Observation with repeat ECHO in 4–6 months

This patient has CREST syndrome and elevated right-sided pulmonary pressures by conventional 2D echocardiogram. Since pulmonary hypertension is a major cause of mortality in these patients, further investigations are warranted. Her Echocardiogram reveals pulmonary hypertension (normal mean PA pressure <25 mmHg) although there is a clear disconnect between her symptoms, examination, and the echo findings. There are differing opinions in this scenario but in an asymptomatic patient she could probably be observed for clinical deterioration or symptoms. A 6-min walk test is also helpful and if abnormal, a right heart catheterization can be considered. This patient had normal PA pressures on right heart catheterization. This case illustrates the limitations of accuracy of echocardiography in obese patients [2, 3, 4].

Answer 103: Posterior reversible encephalopathy syndrome

Posterior reversible encephalopathy syndrome (PRES) or reversible posterior leuko-encephalopathy syndrome (RPLS) is an increasingly recognized neurologic disorder with characteristic computed tomographic (CT) and magnetic resonance (MR) imaging findings, and is associated with a multitude of diverse clinical entities. These include acute glomerulonephritis, preeclampsia and eclampsia, systemic lupus erythematosus, thrombotic thrombocytopenic purpura, and hemolytic-uremic syndrome, as well as drug toxicity from agents such as cyclosporine, tacrolimus, cisplatin, and erythropoietin. Most, but not all, cases manifest with acute to subacute hypertension, and seizures are also frequent. Two pathophysiologic mechanisms for PRES have been proposed. One postulates cerebral vasospasm with resulting ischemia within the involved territories, whereas the other posits a breakdown in cerebrovascular autoregulation with ensuing interstitial extravasation of fluid.

This case is particularly difficult in that a patient with SLE who presents with a seizure and hypertension has to be excluded for active cerebritis or nephritis. The normal lumbar puncture and characteristic MRI findings are highly suggestive of PRES. Treatment involves normalization of BP, removing offending agents such as cytoxan, and prevention of further seizures [5, 6].

Answer 104: Psoriatic arthritis (PsA)

Cutaneous manifestations of psoriasis include oil spots or "oil droplets"—orange-brown patches seen through the nail plate, nail pitting, onycholysis, and subungual hyperkeratosis. Psoriatic nail disease is often associated with psoriatic arthropathy. This patient also has evidence of inflammatory low back pain, uveitis, and sacroiliitis, which are all characteristic of PsA. FABER's test (flexion, abduction, external rotation) is a test for the sacroiliac joint and hip disease. If the patient has pain in the groin it suggests hip pathology but if the pain is in the sacroiliac area it is more consistent with sacroiliitis [7–9].

Answer 105: Large vessel vasculitis
This patient has a recent diagnosis of PMR and now presents with claudication of the left upper extremity in the setting of an absent pulse and markedly elevated inflammatory markers. At this point the diagnosis of exclusion is temporal arteritis (TA) with large vessel involvement. The presence of a subclavian bruit also suggests proximal occlusion. Takayasu's arteritis is also a possibility but less likely given the patient's age and ethnicity. Atherosclerosis needs to be considered but again should not be associated with this degree of inflammation. Large-vessel involvement in giant cell arteritis occurs in over a quarter of patients with this disease. Stenosis of the primary and secondary branches of the aorta may cause claudication and tissue gangrene, whereas aortitis may lead to aneurysm formation and dissection, often many years after the initial diagnosis. The important thing here is to treat the inflammation and ensure that no other organs are involved. A temporal artery biopsy is the best next step. Occasionally TA can be silent and only becomes apparent when a biopsy is performed [10, 11].

Answer 106: Psoriatic arthritis with arthritis mutilans
This is a very destructive form of psoriatic arthritis with significant periarticular bone resorption. The erosions can cause a "pencil in cup" deformity where one articular surface is eroded creating a pointed appearance; the articulating bone can be concave, resembling an upside down cup.

Answer 107: Paget's disease
Diffuse involvement of the left hemipelvis is manifested by areas of mixed sclerosis and lucency. There is also involvement of the right hemipelvis near the right sacroiliac joint, secondary hip osteoarthritis, and thickening of the iliopectineal line.

Antiresorptive treatment should be commenced prior to hip replacement to decrease the hypervascularity and decrease the risk of perioperative bleeding.

Answer 108: Osteitis condensans ilii
Osteitis condensans ilii (OCI) is the radiologic appearance of increased sclerosis in the inferior aspect of the body of the iliac bone arising in a triangular configuration from the lateral aspect of the sacroiliac joint (SI). It is seen most commonly in multiparous women, but also in some degenerative conditions. It is merely a benign reflection of bone remodeling with response to stress, but with the increased radiologic density it is indicative of sclerosis. The SI joints themselves are normal or may feature some degenerative—but not inflammatory or erosive—changes. This condition may sometimes be confused with sacroiliitis, but it can be differentiated by its unilateral nature, lack of erosive or other inflammatory features, both locally and in the spine, and the general absence of clinical symptoms.

Answer 109: Kienbock's disease: avascular necrosis of the lunate
Kienbock's disease is breakdown of the lunate bone, a carpal bone in the wrist that articulates with the radius in the forearm. Fragmentation and collapse of the lunate occurs and has classically been attributed to arterial disruption, but may also occur after events that produce venous congestion with elevated interosseous pressure [12].

Answer 110: Heteretopic ossification

Heterotopic ossification (HO) is the abnormal formation of true bone within extraskeletal soft tissues. The etiology is unclear but this condition can complicate bone forming disorders, joint replacement, blunt trauma, and spinal cord injury.

References

1. Johnston CA, Wiley JP, Lindsay DM, Wiseman DA. Iliopsoas bursitisand tendinitis. A review. Sports Med. 1998;25(4):271–83.
2. Denton CP, Cailes JB, Phillips GD, Wells AU, Black CM, Bois RM. Comparison of Doppler echocardiography and right heart catheterization to assess pulmonary hypertensionin systemic sclerosis. Br J Rheumatol. 1997;36(2):239–43.
3. Gurubhagavatula I, Palevsky HI. Pulmonary hypertension in systemic autoimmune disease. Rheum Dis Clin N Am. 1997;23:365–94.
4. Janda S, Shahidi N, Gin K, et al Diagnostic accuracy of echocardiography for pulmonary hypertension: a systematic review and meta-analysis Heart 2011;97:612–622.
5. Kur JK, Esdaile JM. Posterior reversible encephalopathy syndrome – an underrecognized manifestation of systemic lupus erythematosus. J Rheumatol. 2006;33(11):2178–83. Review
6. Ishimori ML, Pressman BD, Wallace DJ, Weisman MH. Posterior reversible encephalopathy syndrome: another manifestation of CNS SLE? Lupus. 2007;16(6):436–43. Review
7. Paiva ES, Macaluso DC, Edwards A, Rosenbaum JT. Characterisation of uveitisin patients with psoriatic arthritis. Ann Rheum Dis. 2000;59(1):67–70.
8. Turkiewicz AM, Moreland LW. Psoriatic arthritis: current concepts on pathogenesis-oriented therapeutic options. Arthritis Rheum. 2007;56(4):1051–66. Review
9. Zeboulon N, Dougados M, Gossec L. Prevalence and characteristics of uveitisin spondylarthropathies: a systematic literature review. Ann Rheum Dis. 2008;67:955–9.
10. Bongartz T, Matteson EL. Large-vessel involvement in giant cell arteritis. Curr Opin Rheumatol. 2006;18(1):10–7. Review
11. Kwon CM, Hong YH, Chun KA, Cho IH, Kim MJ, Shin DG, Hyun MS, Kim YJ. A case of silent giant cell arteritis involving the entire aorta, carotid artery, and brachial artery screened by integrated PET/CT. Clin Rheumatol. 2007;26(11):1959–62.
12. Bain GI, Yeo CJ, Morse LP. Kienböck Disease: Recent Advances in the Basic Science, Assessment and Treatment. Hand Surg. 2015;20(3):352–65

Chapter 12
Questions 111–120

© Springer International Publishing AG, part of Springer Nature 2018   157
Y. Ali, *Self Assessment in Rheumatology*,
https://doi.org/10.1007/978-3-319-89393-8_12

Question 111

A 55-year-old male has refractory low back pain alleviated by swimming.

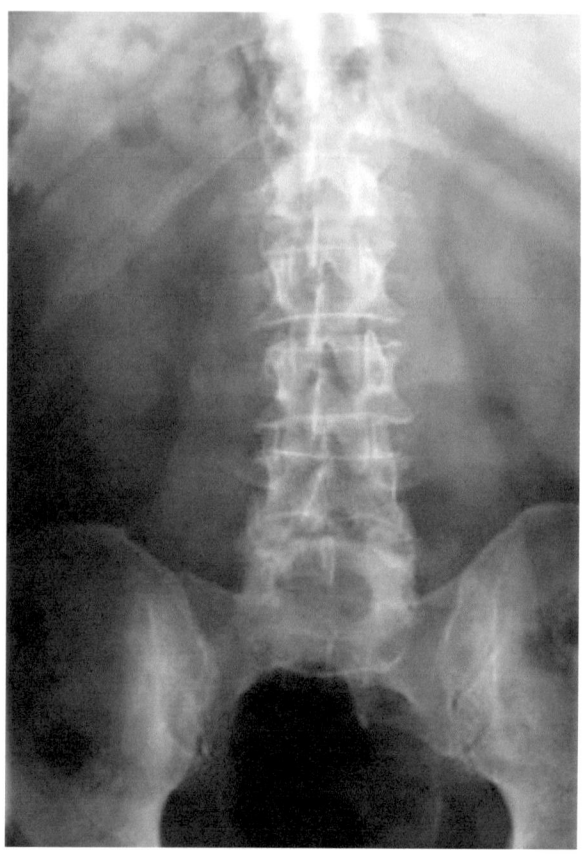

What does the pelvic film show?

Question 112

A 32-year-old male weightlifter has right shoulder pain.

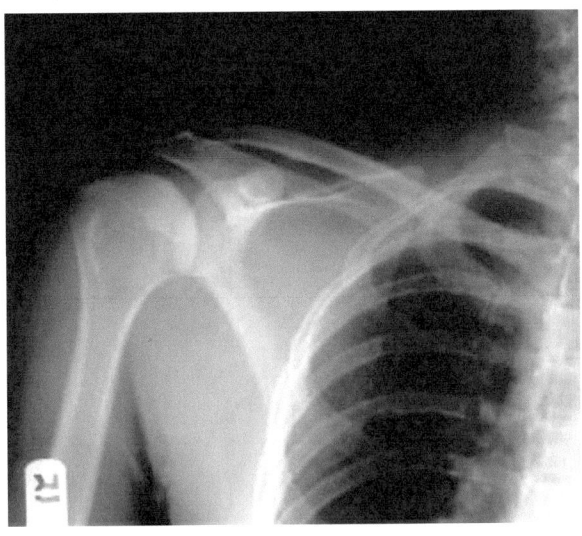

What does the X-ray show?

Question 113

You and a Dermatologist are referred a 45-year-old male to evaluate possible Behcet's syndrome. He has had mucositis for the past month but no fevers, weight loss, uveitis or rash. Apart from his oral findings his exam is normal. Specifically, there are no genital lesions, erythema nodosum or pathergy. Lab data is unremarkable other than the presence of antibodies to desmoglein 1 and 3. The skin biopsy is pending.

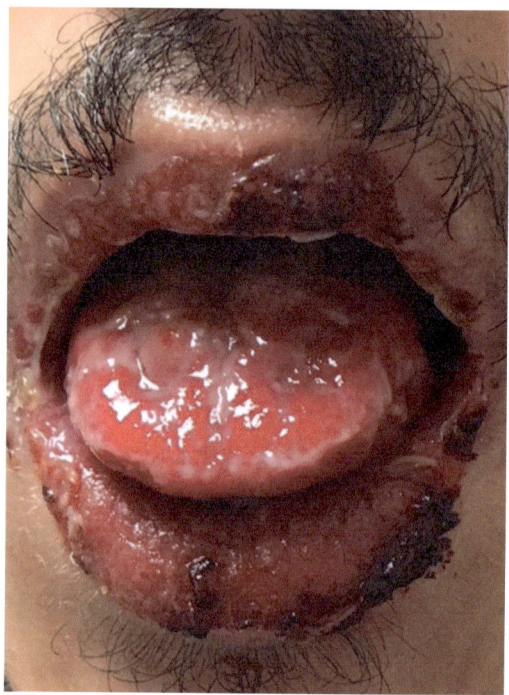

What is the most likely diagnosis?

Question 114

This elderly female has osteoporosis and new pelvic pain.

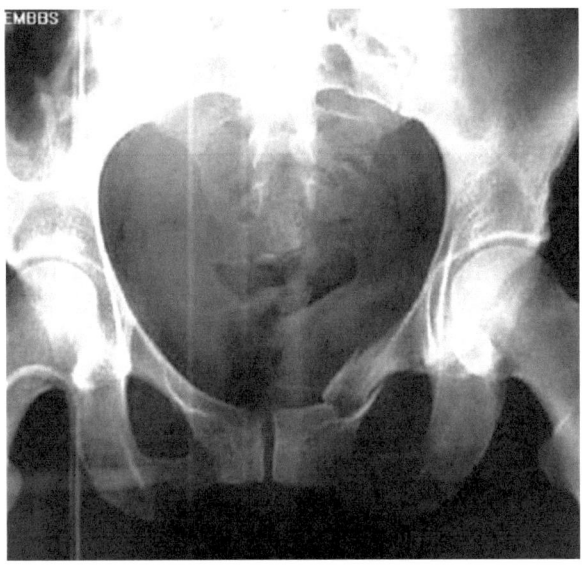

What is the diagnosis?

Question 115

This 45-year-old male has 5 years of RA controlled on Hydroxychloroquine (plaquenil).

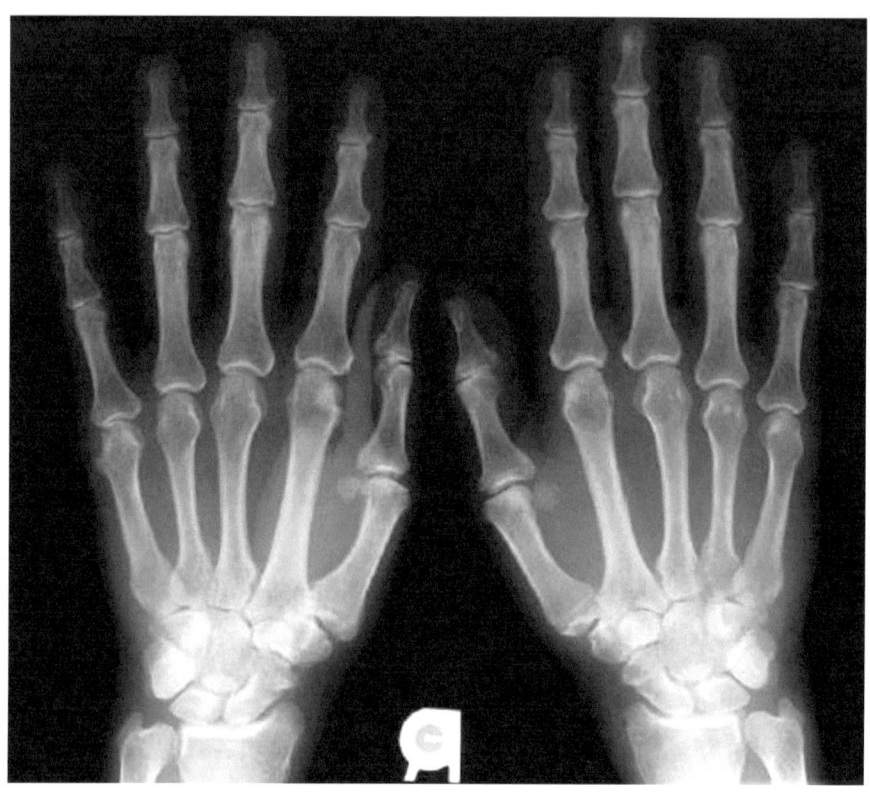

What does his X-ray show?
What would you advise him?

Question 116
This elderly female has sudden onset of excruciating shoulder pain.

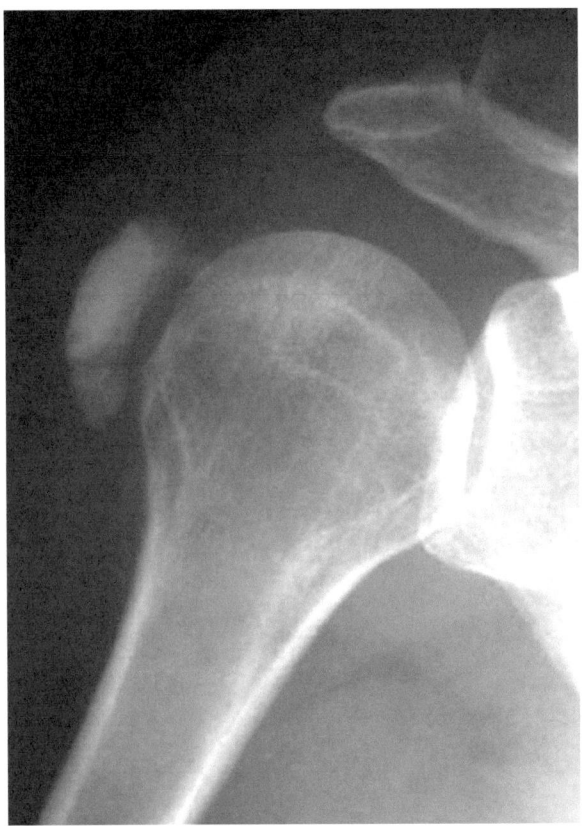

What is the diagnosis?

Question 117

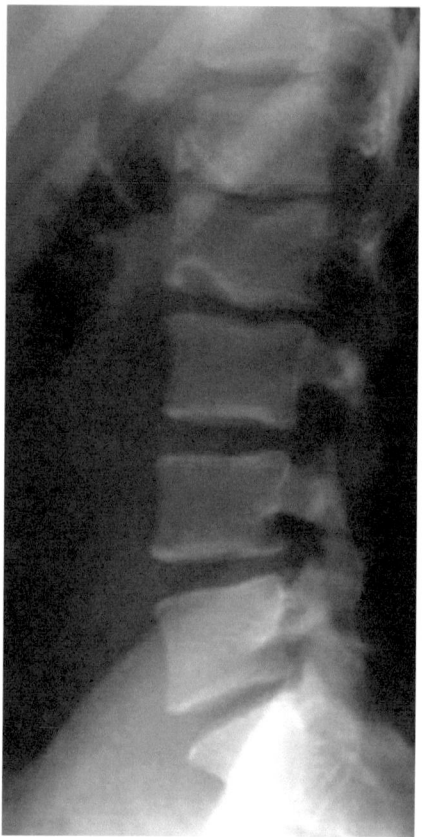

Describe this X-ray.

Question 118

This 77-year-old male is asymptomatic. A routine chest radiograph notes an abnormality in the spine. His lab work is normal.

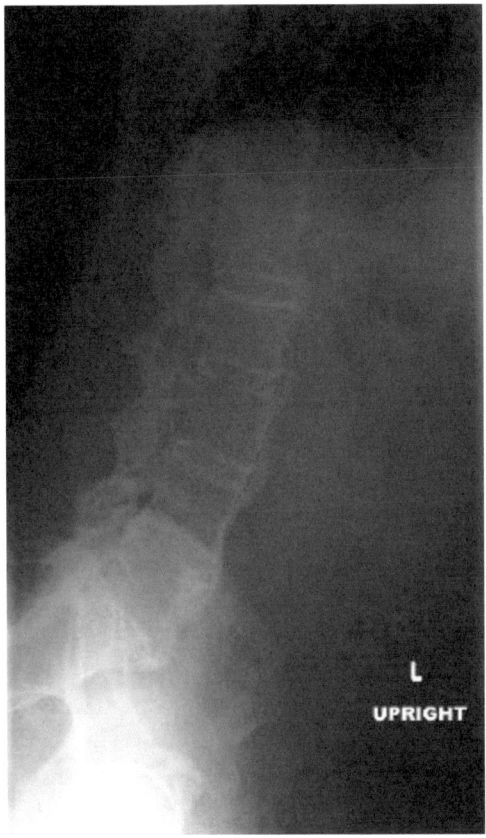

What is the most likely diagnosis based on this lateral view?
What other film would be helpful?
How would you manage him?

Question 119

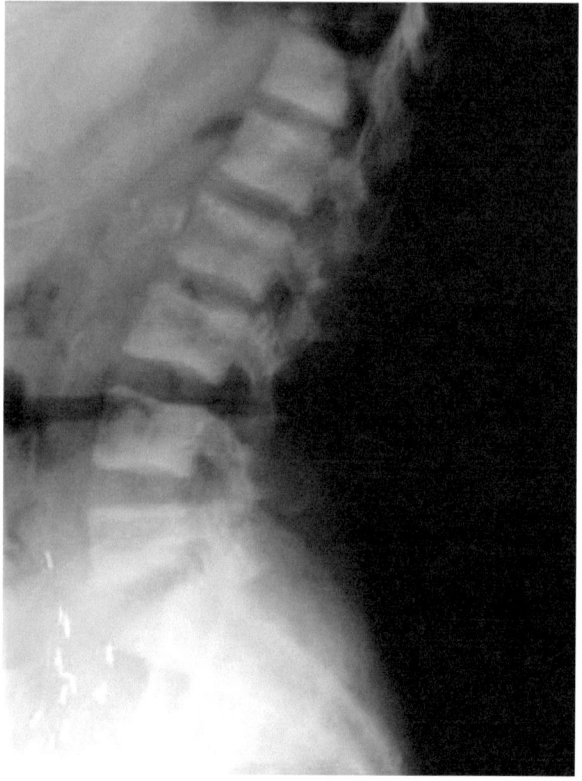

Describe these X-rays.
What is the diagnosis?

Question 120

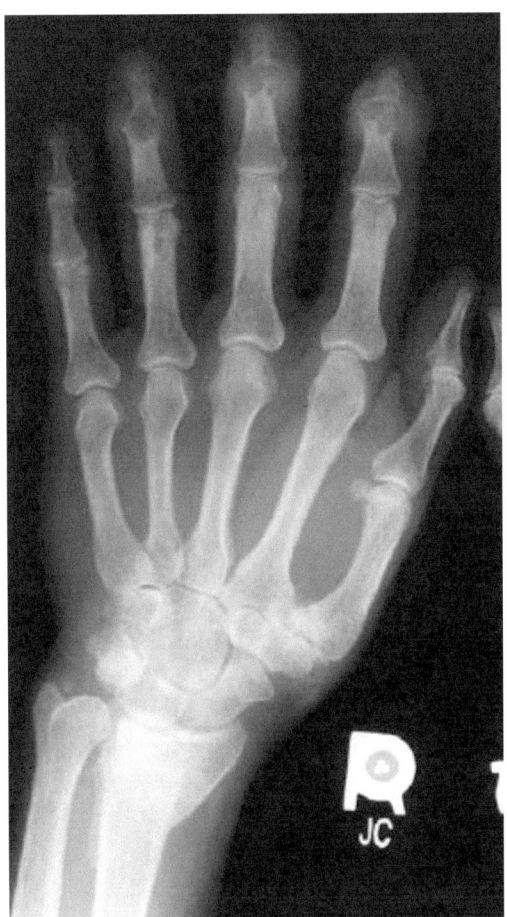

Describe the X-ray.
What is the diagnosis?

Answer 111: Right sacroiliac fusion consistent with a spondyloarthropathy

Answer 112: Right distal clavicleosteolysis induced by weightlifting

Answer 113: Pemphigus Vulgaris (PV)

This condition is a rare autoimmune disease characterized by autoantibodies to desmoglein 1 and 3, mucositis, blistering and oral erosions. Although the differential diagnosis is broad and includes viral associated infection, paraneopastic syndrome and Erythema Multiforme; the presence of these autoantibodies makes PV more likely [1].

Answer 114: Insufficiency fracture of the superior pubic ramus

Answer 115: An erosion at the right fifth MCP joint

A discussion should be had about more aggressive remittive therapy

Answer 116: Calcific tendonitis

This is a disorder characterized by deposits of hydroxyapatite (a crystalline calcium phosphate) in any tendon of the body, but most commonly in the tendons of the rotator cuff (shoulder), causing pain and inflammation.

Answer 117: Schmorl's node at L2

Schmorl's nodes are defined as herniations of the intervertebral disc through the vertebral end-plate. Schmorl's nodes are common, especially with minor degeneration of the aging spine. Schmorl's nodes usually cause no symptoms, but reflect that *wear and tear* of the spine has occurred over time. This radiograph also shows a defect at the anterior body of L1 reflecting protrusion of the intervertebral disk beneath the ring apophysis of the growing vertebral body.

Answer 118: Diffuse skeletal hyperostosis (DISH) syndrome

A pelvic/sacroiliac view would be helpful to exclude sacroiliitis. AS is very unlikely at this age. See Q68 in Chap. 7.

No treatment is indicated

Answer 119: Renal osteodystrophy with Rugger jersey spine. Note the renal transplant

Renal osteodystrophy combines features of secondary hyperparathyroidism, rickets, osteomalacia, and osteoporosis. Bone resorption in renal osteodystrophy is quite complex. Renal retention of phosphate results in hyperphosphatemia, which reduces serum ionized calcium levels, therefore inducing hyperparathyroidism. The hyperparathyroidism increases bone resorption, which may normalize serum calcium levels by releasing the osseous storage of calcium. The various sites of bone resorption include the subperiosteal region of the phalanges, the phalangeal tufts, proximal femur, proximal tibia, proximal humerus, distal clavicle, and calvarial trabeculae. If parathormone levels are mildly elevated over a longer period of time, its effect on bone tends to be anabolic. These effects include excessive maturation of osteoblasts leading to new bone formation and increased laying down of osteoid, which calcifies under the influence of secondarily elevated serum calcium levels. This patient has classic endplate involvement, which results in the appearance of a "Rugger jersey."

Answer 120: Gout with erosions
Characteristic radiographic findings of gout are well-defined, punched-out erosions with overhanging edges, preservation of the joint space, lack of periarticular osteopenia, asymmetrical involvement, soft tissue nodules, and intraosseous calcifications.

Reference

1. Venugopal SS, Murrell DF. Diagnosis and clinical features of pemphigus vulgaris. Immunol Allergy Clin North Am. 2012;32(2):233–43. v–vi.

Index

© Springer International Publishing AG, part of Springer Nature 2018
Y. Ali, *Self Assessment in Rheumatology*,
https://doi.org/10.1007/978-3-319-89393-8

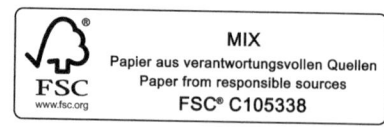

MIX
Papier aus verantwortungsvollen Quellen
Paper from responsible sources
FSC® C105338

If you have any concerns about our products,
you can contact us on
ProductSafety@springernature.com

In case Publisher is established outside the EU,
the EU authorized representative is:
Springer Nature Customer Service Center GmbH
Europaplatz 3, 69115 Heidelberg, Germany

Printed by Libri Plureos GmbH
in Hamburg, Germany